HOW TO START A GARDEN

Turn Your Outdoor Space into a Thriving Oasis

Jeanelle K. Douglas

Contents

INTRODUCTION

Whether you're a beginner or an experienced gardener trying to improve your abilities, this book is your thorough guide to growing your own green sanctuary. Gardening is more than a pastime; it's a journey of discovery, a connection to nature, and a source of fresh, healthy vegetables.

In this book, we'll look at the fundamentals of gardening, its advantages, and what you can expect to learn from this book. Gardening is more than simply planting seeds and watering them; it's a multifaceted process that entails recognizing your surroundings, nurturing plants, and creating a flourishing ecosystem. From choosing the correct plants for your space to dealing with pests and diseases, this book covers every element of gardening, allowing you to begin on this rewarding path with confidence.

We'll go over the essentials of gardening, such as soil preparation, plant selection, and correct maintenance procedures. You'll learn how to design your garden layout, select the finest tools and equipment, and decide whether to start with seeds or seedlings. We'll also look at advanced strategies like companion planting and sustainable gardening practices to help you get the most out of your garden while reducing environmental impact. Whether you envision a rich flower garden, a bountiful vegetable patch, or a tranquil herb garden, "How to Start a Garden" will provide you with the information and skills you need to make your dream a reality. So roll up your sleeves, grab your trowel, and let's embark on this green-fingered journey together.

CHAPTER 1

Understanding the fundamentals of gardening

Gardening is a timeless practice that people have appreciated for generations. At its foundation, gardening is the cultivation of plants for a variety of reasons, including beauty, nourishment, and health. It is a harmonic combination of art, science, and environmental responsibility. Gardening is fundamentally a rewarding pastime that allows people to interact with nature on a deep level. It provides a haven away from the rush and bustle of modern life, providing a peaceful environment for reflection and refreshment. Furthermore, gardening provides a real opportunity to positively impact the environment, whether by supporting local ecosystems with native plantings or lowering one's carbon footprint with produced products.

The benefits of gardening go far beyond the act of planting and caring for plants. Studies have scientifically shown that gardening offers numerous physical, mental, and emotional benefits. Gardening tasks such as digging, planting, and weeding provide beneficial exercise for cardiovascular health, muscle strength, and flexibility. Spending time in the garden lowers stress, anxiety, and depression symptoms, promoting a sense of calm and well-being.

Gardening encourages social contact and community participation. Whether via shared gardening plots, neighborhood garden tours, or community cleaning activities, gardening has the unique capacity to bring people together, forming relationships and instilling a sense of belonging.

Gardening also provides excellent possibilities for intergenerational learning and knowledge sharing, as experienced gardeners pass on their expertise to subsequent generations.

Gardening involves a wide range of activities and traditions, each influenced by cultural history and the geographical climate. From the perfectly groomed gardens of English estates to the lively terraced gardens of the Mediterranean, gardening takes many shapes all over the world.

Also, it is a dynamic and ever-changing activity, with new techniques, equipment, and plant types emerging to fit gardeners' wants and preferences.

Before beginning a gardening adventure, it is critical to examine many important variables that will influence the success and enjoyment of the venture.

These factors include the local temperature and microclimate, soil quality and composition, sunshine exposure, water availability, and one's own time and devotion to the garden. Gardeners may set themselves up for success by carefully examining and arranging these variables, resulting in healthy, sustainable gardens that bring joy and beauty into their lives.

What is gardening?

Gardening is an ancient and very human behavior that entails the intentional nurturing of plants for a number of reasons. Gardening is fundamentally an expression of our instinctive connection to nature. It is an art form that allows people to interact with the environment by molding and nurturing biological creatures to generate beauty, nourishment, and refuge. In its most basic form, gardening is placing seeds or young plants in the soil, giving them the care and resources they require to develop and thrive, and reaping the benefits of one's efforts.

Gardening, on the other hand, includes a wide variety of activities and practices, such as developing and planning garden layouts, selecting appropriate plant species, monitoring soil health, and dealing with pest and disease challenges. Gardening is not just a utilitarian task but also a highly satisfying and rewarding one. It provides a unique chance for people to interact with the natural environment on a personal level, cultivating a sense of connection, wonder, and planet stewardship.

Gardening allows individuals to watch the delicate cycles of the seasons, witness the wondrous process of plant growth and reproduction, and feel the joy of nurturing life. Furthermore, gardening is a multidimensional effort that serves several objectives and meets a wide range of demands. For some, gardening is a kind of creative expression, allowing them to create visually attractive landscapes rich in color, texture, and aroma. Others see gardening as a way to provide food and nourishment, with cultivated fruits, vegetables, and herbs being important components of a healthy diet. Gardening is also very culturally and spiritually significant for many cultures throughout the world.

Traditions, rituals, and ceremonies strongly honor the natural cycles of life and the abundance of the soil. Gardening, whether via community gardening efforts, agricultural-themed religious festivals, or the transmission of gardening expertise from one generation to the next, is a strong symbol of continuity, connection, and resilience. Gardening is a deeply human pursuit that spans time, culture, and country.

It is a timeless practice that expresses our underlying need to nurture and cultivate life, to produce beauty and plenty, and to form meaningful connections with the natural world and one another. Gardening provides a retreat in an increasingly fast-paced and disconnected society, allowing us to reconnect with the cycles of nature, build a sense of purpose and belonging, and find peace and refreshment for the mind, body, and soul.

Benefits of Gardening

Gardening has several advantages that go well beyond the basic act of planting and caring for plants. Gardening activities may have a significant positive impact on physical health, emotional well-being, and social relationships. Gardening is a great way to get some good exercise and improve your cardiovascular health, muscle strength, and flexibility.

Digging, planting, weeding, and watering all involve physical labor, which helps to increase general fitness and contributes to a healthy lifestyle.

Spending time outside in the fresh air and sunshine gives you much-needed vitamin D, which is required for bone health and immunological function.

Gardening offers considerable mental health benefits. Working with plants and soil has the potential to be naturally therapeutic, lowering stress, anxiety, and depression symptoms.

Gardening provides a sense of purpose and success as people see the results of their efforts develop and blossom. The act of caring for live creatures generates a sense of connectedness to nature, which promotes awareness, tranquility, and well-being.

Gardening allows for essential social connections and community participation. Gardening has the unique capacity to bring people together, develop ties, and create a feeling of belonging.

Gardening also provides possibilities for intergenerational learning and information sharing, as experienced gardeners pass on their expertise to subsequent generations.

Gardening may have a positive environmental impact by increasing biodiversity, sequestering carbon, and improving ecosystem health. Gardeners may help to sustain local ecosystems and preserve native species by cultivating native plants and building wildlife-friendly habitats.

Homegrown fruits, vegetables, and herbs lower the carbon footprint associated with food production and transportation, resulting in increased sustainability and resilience in the face of climate change.

Gardening is a deeply gratifying and rewarding pastime that provides several physical, mental, and social advantages. Whether you have a large backyard garden or a few pots on a windowsill, gardening may improve your quality of life, increase well-being, and develop relationships with nature and others.

Types of Gardens

Gardening involves a wide range of activities and traditions, each influenced by cultural history and the geographical climate. From the perfectly groomed gardens of English estates to the lively terraced gardens of the Mediterranean, gardening takes many shapes all over the world.

Ornamental gardens: They are undoubtedly the most well-known, valued for their aesthetic beauty and visual appeal. Expertly organized blooming plants, shrubs, and trees in these gardens create gorgeous landscapes that please the senses. Whether it's a formal French garden with precisely designed hedges and symmetrical flower beds or a charming cottage garden brimming with brilliant blossoms, ornamental gardens provide limitless opportunities for creative expression.

Vegetable gardens: On the other hand, emphasize utility over appearance, cultivating edible plants for personal use. These gardens can range from little raised beds or containers on a balcony to large areas of ground dedicated to cultivating a diverse range of fruits, vegetables, and herbs.

Vegetable gardening is a wonderful way to reconnect with the origins of our food, encourage sustainability, and enjoy the unique flavor and freshness of homegrown vegetables. Herb gardens provide a unique niche in the gardening world, acting as both functional and ornamental locations.

These gardens have a wide collection of aromatic plants valued for their culinary, medicinal, and fragrant characteristics.

Herb gardens: Provide a plethora of options for cooking, healing, and sensory delight, ranging from traditional culinary herbs like basil, thyme, and rosemary to medicinal herbs like chamomile and Echinacea.

Specialty gardens : Cater to specific hobbies or preferences by displaying distinctive plant collections or design styles. These gardens can take many different shapes, ranging from the peaceful peacefulness of a Japanese Zen garden to the whimsical beauty of a fairy garden.

Specialty gardens can also focus on certain themes or goals, such as rock gardens with drought-tolerant plants, water gardens with aquatic plants and fish, or butterfly gardens that attract and sustain native pollinators. Additional types of gardens that demonstrate the range and depth of gardening practices:

1. Wildlife Gardens: These gardens are specifically intended to attract and sustain local wildlife, including birds, butterflies, bees, and beneficial insects. Animal gardens prioritize native plant species that offer food, shelter, and nesting places for animals, while also including elements such as bird feeders, bee hotels, and water supplies to increase habitat variety.

2. Permaculture Gardens: Permaculture gardens use sustainable design concepts to replicate natural ecosystems and generate productive, self-sustaining systems. These gardens integrate food production, water management, energy efficiency, and waste recycling in a harmonic manner, with the goal of increasing yields while decreasing inputs and environmental effects.

3. Rooftop Gardens: In highly populated metropolitan areas with limited ground space, rooftop gardens provide a unique alternative for urban greening. These gardens use rooftops, balconies, and other high locations to create a green oasis where inhabitants may relax, play, and grow food. Rooftop gardens can also help minimize urban heat island effects, save energy, and enhance air quality.

4. Vertical Gardens: Vertical gardens, often called living walls or green walls, are vertical buildings covered in plants. These gardens make good use of limited space by growing plants vertically on walls, fences, and trellises. Vertical gardens may be both beautiful and practical, offering insulation, noise reduction, and aesthetic appeal in urban settings.

5. Ethnobotanical Gardens: These gardens honor indigenous peoples' cultural legacy and traditional knowledge by displaying plants of historical, medicinal, or ceremonial importance. These gardens serve as living museums, preserving and sharing the rich floral diversity and cultural legacy of many communities around the world. They frequently include interpretive signs, educational activities, and interactive exhibits emphasizing the cultural and ecological significance of native plants.

6. Xeriscapes: Xeriscapes is a landscaping technique that prioritizes water conservation and drought tolerance. These gardens use native or modified plants that are well-suited to local environmental conditions and grow in dry or semi-arid settings with minimal watering. Xeriscapes frequently use water-saving practices like mulching, soil amendment, and efficient irrigation systems to minimize water use and enhance sustainability.

7. Container Gardens: Container gardening is a flexible and space-saving gardening technique that involves growing plants in containers like pots, planters, or raised beds. City residents, renters, and individuals with limited outdoor space can easily plant container gardens on patios, balconies, or windowsills. Container gardens provide flexibility and mobility, allowing gardeners to experiment with different plant combinations and relocate plants as needed to achieve ideal growth conditions.

These additional types of gardens demonstrate the wide diversity of gardening methods and approaches that appeal to a variety of interests, surroundings, and lifestyles. Whether you want to attract animals, maximize sustainability, or make the most of limited space, there is a gardening style to meet your requirements and interests.

Chapter 2

Factors to Consider Before venturing into the wonderful world of gardening

You should take some time to evaluate many crucial elements that will impact the success and satisfaction of your gardening pursuits. First and foremost, evaluate your local climate and environmental factors.

Understanding your climatic zone will help you choose plants that thrive in your area's temperature ranges, rainfall patterns, and seasonal fluctuations. Consider typical temperatures, frost dates, and precipitation amounts to ensure your garden thrives in its environment.

Then, assess the available area for your garden. Whether you have a large backyard, a small balcony, or even a sunny windowsill, it's critical to select plants and gardening techniques that are fit for your space limits. When designing the layout and style of your garden, take into account aspects such as sunlight exposure, soil quality, and water availability.

Soil quality is another important concern when developing a garden. Take the time to analyze the composition and condition of your soil, since it has a direct influence on plant development and output. Before planting, assess your soil's pH, texture, and nutrient levels to see if any changes or enhancements are required. Consider adding organic matter, such as compost or old manure, to increase soil structure and fertility.

In addition to the soil condition, think about the availability of water in your garden. Evaluate your water supply options and, if required, construct irrigation or rainfall gathering equipment. Consider water-saving methods and select drought-tolerant plants that need less water to grow in your garden. Another key element to consider is your time and dedication to the garden.

Gardening needs regular maintenance duties such as watering, weeding, and trimming, so it's critical to estimate how much time you can devote to caring for your plants. Begin small and gradually grow your garden as you become familiar with the upkeep requirements.

When planting and developing your garden, keep your gardening goals and tastes in mind. Whether you want to cultivate flowers, veggies, herbs, or a combination of the three, select plants that match your hobbies and gardening style. Consider plant size, growth habit, and bloom period when designing a garden that matches your unique style and aesthetic preferences.

Plan Your Garden Plan your garden

Planning your garden ahead of time may considerably improve its success and enjoyment. Garden planning entails carefully considering a variety of aspects, including analyzing your area, selecting appropriate plants, and developing the layout. By following a methodical planning approach, you can design a garden that fulfills your needs, expresses your own style, and thrives throughout the year.

Begin by evaluating your available area and determining its unique traits. Make a note of the size, shape, and orientation of your garden, as well as any existing elements like trees, structures, or obstructions. Consider elements like sunlight exposure, soil quality, and drainage patterns, since these will all impact plant choices and location. Next, determine your gardening goals and priorities.

Are you primarily interested in producing flowers, veggies, herbs, or a mix of the three?

Do you want to build a peaceful refuge for leisure, a lively spot for partying, or a productive garden for growing food?

Clarifying your goals can help you make plant selection and design decisions.

Once you've determined your area and goals, it's time to select the appropriate plants for your garden. When choosing plants that are most suited to your location, keep your local climate, soil conditions, and available sunshine in mind. Investigate several plant varieties to determine their growth requirements, care requirements, and suitability for your garden settings.

With your plant choices in mind, it's time to arrange the layout of your garden. When placing plants in your garden beds or containers, consider their size, growth habits, and spacing needs. Consider adding components like walkways, focal spots, and seating places to improve the usefulness and visual appeal of your garden. Use color, texture, and contrast to add visual appeal to your garden arrangement.

Experiment with various plant combinations and arrangements to achieve dynamic and harmonic ensembles. Consider layering, grouping, and repetition to provide depth and consistency to your garden design.

While finalizing your garden layout, keep practical considerations like irrigation, mulching, and care in mind.

Make sure your garden plan provides for easy access to water sources and maintenance jobs, and think about including sustainable techniques like water-efficient irrigation systems and organic mulches to enhance soil health and preserve resources. By properly designing your garden, you may create a beautiful, practical, and long-lasting outdoor space that will provide you with joy and contentment for many years.

Whether you're beginning from scratch or redesigning an existing garden, taking the time to plan carefully can set you up for success in your gardening activities.

Assessing Your Space

Assessing your space before you start designing and planting your garden

You need to carefully examine your available area. Understanding the specific qualities of your garden can allow you to make more educated judgments regarding plant selection, layout, and design.

Here are some important factors to consider while appraising your space:

1. Size and form: Measure your garden's measurements to determine its size and form. Consider the overall area available for gardening, as well as any specialized parts or zones within the space. Take note of any abnormalities or barriers in your garden plan, such as slopes, curves, or awkward corners. Determine the direction of your garden space and how much sunshine it receives throughout the day.

2. Exposure: Determine the direction of your garden space and how much sunshine it receives throughout the day. Make a note of any spots that receive full sun, medium shade, or deep shadow; these will impact your plant choices. Keep in mind that sunlight patterns might alter throughout the seasons depending on factors such as the sun's location and the existence of adjacent structures or trees.

3. Soil Quality: Evaluate your soil's fertility, texture, and drainage properties. Take a soil sample and do a basic soil test to evaluate pH and nutrient content. Identify any issues like compacted soil, poor drainage, or nutrient shortages that require attention before planting.

4. Existing Features: Take note of any existing features in your garden, such as trees, bushes, buildings, or hardscape pieces. Think about incorporating these elements into your garden design or how they might influence plant choices and placement. When planning your garden layout, consider elements like root competition, shade, and sight lines.

5. Microclimates: Identify any sections of your garden that are unusually hot, chilly, windy, or protected. The proximity of buildings, fences, or bodies of water can all have an impact on these microclimates. Consider how various microclimates may influence plant development, and select plants that are best suited to their individual environmental circumstances.

6. Accessibility: Consider the accessibility of your garden space, as well as how it will affect your ability to care for your plants and perform maintenance duties. Ensure that routes are broad enough for simple access and that no impediments or dangers obstruct mobility. Consider adding elements like raised beds or container gardens to make gardening more accessible to those with mobility challenges. Before you begin gardening, properly examine your space.

This will allow you to make educated decisions and design a garden that thrives in its surroundings. Taking the time to learn your garden's particular traits can set you up for success and make gardening pleasurable and gratifying.

Choosing the Appropriate Location

Choosing the best site for your garden is an important step toward ensuring its success and output. The appropriate location may create perfect circumstances for plant development while mitigating issues like poor soil quality and insufficient sunshine.

Here are some aspects to consider while choosing the best site for your garden:

1. Sunshine Exposure: Most plants require plenty of sunshine to grow, so select a site that receives plenty of sunlight throughout the day. Observe your garden area at various times of day to determine the quantity and intensity of sunshine it gets. Most vegetables, herbs, and floral plants benefit from at least six to eight hours of direct sunshine every day.

2. Soil quality: has a substantial impact on plant development and production. Conduct a soil test to determine your soil's pH, nutritional content, and texture. Choose a place with well-drained soil high in organic matter and nutrients. If your soil is of low quality, consider adding compost, organic matter, or soil amendments to increase its fertility and structure.

3. Water Availability: Make sure your preferred site has access to water for irrigation purposes. Consider the proximity of water sources such as outdoor faucets, rainwater collection systems, and irrigation systems. Choose a place that provides for easy irrigation equipment installation and uniform water delivery to your plants.

 4. Be conscious of microclimates in your garden, which are small-scale differences in temperature, humidity, and wind patterns. The proximity of buildings, fences, or bodies of water can all have an impact on these microclimates. Choose a place with little exposure to severe temperatures, strong winds, and other hazardous environmental factors.

5. Space and Layout: When deciding where to put your garden, keep its design in mind. Make sure that the chosen area has adequate room for your desired garden size and style, including walkways, beds, and other elements. Choose a place that provides for simple access and transit within the garden, as well as ample room for planting, harvesting, and upkeep.

6. Visual Considerations: Consider the visual attractiveness of your garden placement and how it will work with your overall landscape plan. Select a location that enhances the visual appeal of your outdoor area and fosters a unified and harmonious environment. When deciding where to plant your garden, consider vistas, sight lines, and focus points. By carefully examining these aspects while selecting the best site for your garden, you can create an ideal growing environment that promotes plant health, production, and overall satisfaction. Taking the effort to choose the ideal place can pave the way for a successful and satisfying gardening experience for years to come.

Chapter 3

Selecting Plants

Selecting Plants Choosing the proper plants for your garden is critical to establishing a healthy and attractive outdoor area. Whether you want to produce flowers, veggies, herbs, or a combination of the three, choosing plants that are appropriate for your climate, soil, and growth conditions is critical to success. When picking plants for your garden, consider the following factors:

1. Consider your local temperature and hardiness zone: Choose plants that are well-suited to your area's temperature, rainfall, and frost patterns. Consult a hardiness zone chart to identify which plants are appropriate for your location and select types that have proven to survive in your unique climate circumstances.

 2. Sunlight Requirements: Determine the quantity of sunlight available in your garden and select plants that meet its requirements. Some plants like direct sunlight, while others flourish in moderate or deep shadow. Take notice of your garden's direction and how lighting patterns change throughout the day to ensure that your chosen plants receive an adequate quantity of light.

3. Soil type and pH: When choosing plants for your garden, keep your soil's type and pH in mind. Some plants favor acidic soils, while others flourish in alkaline or neutral soil. Conduct a soil test to assess your soil's pH level, and select plants that thrive in its acidity or alkalinity. Consider soil texture as well, and select plants that are appropriate for your soil's drainage and structure.

4. Water Requirements: To facilitate effective irrigation and water management in your garden, select plants with comparable water requirements. Some plants are drought-tolerant and need little watering, but others are water-intensive and require frequent irrigation. Consider your garden's availability of water sources and select plants that are suitable for your watering schedule and conservation objectives.

5. Growth Habit and Size: When designing your garden layout, keep your plants' growth habits and sizes in mind. Choose plants that are appropriate for the size and proportions of your garden space, avoiding overcrowding or competition for resources. Consider plant height, spread, and growth rate to ensure that your garden design is harmonious and balanced.

6. Seasonal Interest: Choose plants that add interest and beauty throughout the year to create a dynamic and visually pleasing landscape. Choose a variety of plants with varying bloom periods, leaf colors, and textures to offer year-round pleasure. Consider using seasonal annuals, perennials, and evergreens to create a garden that grows and changes with the seasons.

7. Pest and Disease Resistance: Choose plants that are resistant to the most prevalent pests and diseases in your region to reduce the need for chemical treatments and care. Investigate plant types noted for their pest and disease resistance, and select cultivars that are well-suited to your garden's growing circumstances. By carefully considering these aspects when choosing plants for your garden, you can build a diversified and resilient outdoor environment that flourishes throughout the year. Take the time to study and select plants that are appropriate for your climate, soil, and growth conditions, and you will be able to enjoy the beauty and fullness of your garden for many years.

Plan Your Garden Layout

Layout designing your garden layout is a creative and satisfying process that allows you to convert your outside area into a beautiful and useful sanctuary. Whether you're beginning from scratch or remodeling an existing garden, careful planning is required to create a place that represents your own style, fits your gardening requirements, and increases your love of the outdoors.

When developing your garden layout, consider the following steps:

1. Assess Your Space: Start by determining the size, shape, and characteristics of your garden space. Take measurements and draw a rough sketch or map of the site, noting any existing components such as trees, structures, or walkways. Consider incorporating these characteristics into your garden design, or consider how they may affect the layout of your beds and walkways.

2. Define Your Garden Zones: Divide your garden into various zones or sections depending on your gardening objectives and preferences. Consider making distinct zones for different sorts of plants, such as flowers, vegetables, herbs, and decorative shrubs. Set aside room for useful items like lounging places, compost bins, and tool sheds. Define precise borders between each zone to provide visual separation and organization in your garden.

3. Plan Your Beds and Borders: Choose the placement and arrangement of your garden beds and borders for each zone. When arranging your beds, take into account solar exposure, soil quality, and water availability. Experiment with different forms, sizes, and layouts to add interest and diversity to your landscape. Allow enough room between beds for paths, access, and future plant growth.

4. Choose plants that are appropriate for your climate, soil, and growth circumstances. When picking plants for each bed or border, keep sunshine, water requirements, and mature size in mind. Aim for a variety of colors, textures, and heights to create a visually pleasing and dynamic garden

design. Group plants with comparable care requirements together to make upkeep and watering easier.

5. Design your paths: Create paths and walkways to allow access and circulation around your garden. Consider traffic flow, accessibility, and safety while constructing walkways. Use gravel, paving stones, or mulch to delineate walkways and provide visual interest. Experiment with various forms and patterns to give your landscape design uniqueness and charm.

6. Incorporate Hardscape Elements: Add garden structures, raised beds, trellises, or water features to your garden design. These elements may offer vertical interest, structure, and focus points to your garden while also improving its usefulness and attractiveness. Choose materials and designs that complement your garden's aesthetic and work well with the surrounding surroundings.

7. Add Finishing Touches: Once you've decided on your garden layout, add finishing touches like ornamental accents, garden art, or container plantings to enhance the beauty and uniqueness of your outdoor space. Consider adding sitting spaces, lights, or other amenities to extend the use of your garden into the evening. Color, texture, and size are all important things to consider when creating a unified and welcoming garden design. By following these steps and embracing your imagination, you can create a garden layout that reflects your own vision and adds joy and beauty to your outdoor environment. Remember to be adaptable and open to experimenting while you work on your design, and don't be afraid to let your individuality come through in every area of your garden arrangement.

Preparing Your Garden Space

Preparing your garden area is an important step in creating a healthy and productive outdoor paradise. Proper preparation ensures that your soil is healthy and fertile, that your plants have the best possible growing conditions, and that your garden is ready to thrive. Here are some procedures to take when preparing your garden space:

1. Clean the Area: Begin by clearing the garden of any waste, weeds, or unwanted plants. Remove any rocks, sticks, or other objects that may obstruct planting or interfere with gardening operations. To loosen and eliminate weeds, use a rake or garden hoe, taking care to remove the roots to avoid a recurrence.

2. Test the soil: Perform a soil test to determine the pH, nutritional content, and texture of your soil. Soil testing kits are available at garden stores or from your local agricultural extension office. Follow the kit's instructions to gather soil samples from various parts of your garden. Once you have the data, treat your soil as needed to alter pH levels and increase fertility.

3. Improve Soil Structure: Add organic matter like compost, aged manure, or leaf mold to your soil to boost its structure and fertility. Spread a layer of organic matter over the soil's surface and work it in with a garden fork or tiller to a depth of 6–8 inches. Organic matter improves soil drainage, water retention, and nutrient availability, resulting in an optimal environment for plant development.

4. Level the ground: Make sure the ground in your garden is smooth and level before planting. Use a garden rake or leveling tool to remove any high points and fill in any low places. To avoid water gathering, pay attention to drainage patterns and make sure your garden slopes slightly away from structures or low-lying areas.

5. Plan Your Layout: Determine the placement of your garden beds, paths, and other elements within your garden area. When arranging your beds, take into account solar exposure, plant spacing, and access to water supplies. To make it easier to organize and maintain your garden, set distinct boundaries between each region.

6. Install any hardscape elements: such as raised beds, trellises, or garden structures, prior to planting. Use wood, stone, or metal to build long-lasting and visually appealing garden elements. Properly secure and level hardscape features to prevent them from moving or settling over time.

7. Prepare Planting Beds: Loosen the soil and add organic materials to produce a nutrient-rich growth environment. Using a garden fork or tiller, loosen the soil to a depth of 6–8 inches, taking care not to compress it. Smooth the bed's surface with a rake and make planting rows or mounds as needed, depending on your planting scheme.

8. Mulch and Protect: Cover the surface of your planting beds with a layer of mulch, such as straw, wood chips, or shredded leaves, to preserve moisture, discourage weeds, and regulate soil temperature. Mulch also helps to prevent soil erosion and compaction, resulting in a healthy and resilient growth environment for your plants. Following these procedures and taking the time to properly prepare your garden space will help you establish an optimal environment for plant development and assure the success of your gardening efforts. Remember to be careful and attentive in your preparations, and enjoy the experience of developing your outside area into a beautiful and productive garden.

CHAPTER 4

Clearing the Area

Cleaning up the area before you can begin developing your fantasy garden, make sure the space is free of waste, weeds, and undesirable plants. Clearing the space completely prepares the ground for effective gardening by creating a clear canvas for planting and reducing competition for resources.

Here's how to efficiently clear the space for your garden:

1. Remove Debris: First, clear the area of any significant debris, such as rocks, branches, or old garden constructions. Clearing these impediments will make it easier to work in the area and reduce tripping hazards while gardening.

2. Weed Removal: Using a garden hoe, rake, or weed trimmer, remove any existing weeds or vegetation from the area. To inhibit regrowth, pluck weeds by their roots. To efficiently eradicate bigger areas or thick weed infestations, employ a weed killer or herbicide.

3. You may need to remove grass, shrubs, or other vegetation with a lawnmower, brush cutter, or chainsaw. Cut down overgrown plants to ground level, and remove any plant debris from the area.

4. Dig out Roots: After cutting down plants, remove any leftover roots or stumps to avoid regrowth. To loosen the dirt surrounding the roots and lift them out of the earth, use a shovel or digging instrument. To avoid future problems with invasive plants, thoroughly remove the roots.

5. Level the Ground: After clearing the trash and weeds, use a rake or leveling tool to smooth and level the ground. To produce a flat and even planting site, remove any residual rocks, dirt clumps, or other obstructions. Remove any debris, plant material, or other garbage created during the clearing procedure. Organic material, such as weeds or grass clippings, may be compostable, but larger garbage may require disposal at a recycling facility or landfill.

6. Protect Surrounding Areas: During the clearance process, take precautions to keep nearby areas, such as adjacent gardens or natural ecosystems, safe from harm. To keep trash from spreading outside the garden area and to reduce disruptions to surrounding plants and wildlife, use barriers or fencing. Before you begin gardening, completely cleanse the area to produce a clean and neat environment suitable for planting and growing. Making the effort to carefully clean the space will pave the way for effective planting and guarantee that your garden flourishes in its new setting.

Soil Preparation

Soil Preparation Preparing the soil is a critical step in growing a healthy and productive garden. Proper soil preparation ensures that your plants have access to the necessary nutrients, adequate drainage, and a favorable growing environment.

Here's how to prepare your soil for successful gardening:

1. Soil Testing: Begin by testing your soil to determine its pH, nutrient content, and texture. Soil testing kits are available at garden stores or from your local agricultural extension office. Follow the kit's instructions to gather soil samples from various parts of your garden. When you receive the results, you'll have valuable information to help you plan your soil preparation efforts.

2. Amend soil pH: Based on the results of your soil test, adjust the pH levels of your soil as necessary. Most plants prefer a slightly acidic to neutral pH, usually between 6.0 and 7.0. If your soil is too acidic (low pH), you can increase its pH by adding lime. If the pH is too high (alkaline), you can lower it by adding sulfur or peat moss.

3. Add Organic Matter: To improve soil structure and fertility, incorporate organic matter such as compost, aged manure, or leaf mold. Spread a layer of organic matter over the soil's surface and work it in with a garden fork or tiller to a depth of 6–8 inches. Organic matter increases soil moisture retention, improves soil aeration, and provides essential nutrients for plant development.

4. Improve Soil Texture: If your soil is heavy clay or compacted, you can improve its texture by adding sand, perlite, or vermiculite. These amendments help to loosen the soil, improve drainage, and provide a more favorable environment for plant roots to grow. Mix the amendments thoroughly into the soil to ensure even distribution across the planting area.

5. Provide Drainage: Make sure your soil has adequate drainage to avoid waterlogging and root rot. If your soil is heavy clay or retains water, add organic matter and amendments to improve drainage. To improve drainage in poor-draining areas, consider installing raised beds or planting on mounds.

6. Remove Weeds and Debris: Prior to planting, clear the soil surface of any weeds, rocks, or debris. Weeds compete with your plants for nutrients and water, so get rid of them before they spread. Remove weeds from the soil surface with a hoe, rake, or by hand.

7. Mulch the Soil: After preparing the soil, spread a layer of mulch, such as straw, wood chips, or shredded leaves, across the surface. Mulch conserves moisture, suppresses weeds, and regulates soil temperatures. Spread a layer of mulch, 2-4 inches thick, over the soil surface, taking care not to pile it against the plant stems. Following these soil preparation steps will result in a healthy and fertile growing environment for your plants. Taking the time to properly prepare the soil will result in healthier plants, increased yields, and a more successful garden overall.

Adding Soil Amendments

Adding soil amendments Soil amendments are beneficial additions to your garden that can enhance soil structure, fertility, and overall plant health. Whether you have sandy soil that drains too quickly or clay soil that retains too much water, adding amendments can help your plants thrive.

Here's how to apply soil amendments effectively:

 1. **Assess Soil Needs:** Before adding any soil amendments, you should first understand your soil's specific requirements. Perform a soil test to determine pH, nutrient deficiencies, and soil texture. This information will help you select appropriate soil amendments and address any deficiencies or imbalances in your soil.

2. **Choose the Right Amendments:** Select soil amendments based on your soil's specific needs and your plants' requirements.

Common soil amendments include the following

Organic Matter: Compost, aged manure, leaf mold, or composted kitchen scraps all contribute valuable organic matter to the soil, improving structure, moisture retention, and nutrient availability.

Lime: Adding lime increases soil pH, making acidic soils more alkaline and less acidic. Farmers frequently use lime to adjust the pH of acidic soils for optimal plant growth.

Sulfur: Sulfur reduces soil pH, making alkaline soils more acidic. Its purpose is to reduce soil alkalinity and create a more acidic environment for acid-loving plants.

Perlite or vermiculite: These lightweight, porous materials enhance soil aeration and drainage, particularly in heavy clay soils. They also help to prevent soil compaction and promote root growth.

3. Apply Amendments: Once you've chosen the appropriate soil amendments, spread them evenly across the soil surface in accordance with the package instructions or recommended application rates. Spread compost or aged manure in a layer several inches thick, then work it into the soil to a depth of 6–8 inches with a garden fork or tiller. For amendments such as lime or sulfur, use the application rates specified on the package based on your soil test results.

4. Incorporate into the soil: After applying soil amendments, thoroughly mix and distribute them throughout the soil. Use a garden fork, hoe, or tiller to incorporate the amendments into the soil to the desired depth. Be careful not to over-till or disturb the soil too much, as this can disrupt soil structure and beneficial soil organisms.

5. Water Thoroughly: After incorporating the soil amendments, water the soil thoroughly to help settle them and promote their integration into the soil. Watering also stimulates microbial activity and initiates the decomposition of organic amendments like compost or manure.

 6. Monitor and Adjust: After adding soil amendments, check your soil on a regular basis to assess its response and make any necessary adjustments. Pay attention to plant growth, soil moisture levels, and nutrient availability to ensure that your soil amendments are having the desired effect. You may need to reapply amendments on a regular basis to keep soil health and fertility stable over time.

Create garden beds or containers

Building garden beds or containers is an important step towards creating a functional and visually appealing garden space. Whether you're growing vegetables, flowers, or herbs, the right containers or raised beds can provide ideal growing conditions while also making gardening more accessible. Here's how to build garden beds or containers efficiently:

1. Choose Your Design: Determine the type and design of garden beds or containers that best meet your gardening requirements and space constraints. Raised beds, container gardens, vertical gardens, and traditional in-ground planting beds are all common options. When deciding on a design, consider available space, sunlight exposure, and personal aesthetic preferences.

2. Choose Materials: When building your garden beds or containers, use materials that are durable and weather-resistant. Common materials include wood (such as cedar or redwood), stone, brick, concrete blocks, plastic, and metal.

Choose materials that are appropriate for your climate and budget, and make sure they are safe to use in gardening applications.

3. Determine the size and dimensions of your garden beds or containers based on available space, plant selection, and accessibility requirements. Raised beds and containers should be wide enough to accommodate your plants' root systems while also providing enough soil depth for healthy growth. Raised beds should be 3–4 feet wide, while containers should be at least 12–18 inches deep.

4. Build Raised Beds: Start by marking the outline of your bed with stakes, string, or a garden hose. Prepare the site by leveling and clearing any debris or vegetation. Assemble the raised bed frame from your chosen materials, securing the corners with screws or brackets. To prevent weeds from growing up into the bed, line the bottom with landscape fabric and fill with a mix of topsoil, compost, and other amendments.

5. Construct Containers: If you're using containers, choose pots or planters that are the right size and materials for your plants. To prevent waterlogging and root rot, ensure that containers have adequate drainage holes in the bottom. Fill the containers with a nutrient-dense, well-drained potting mix or container soil. To improve drainage, consider adding a layer of gravel or broken pottery shards to the bottom of larger containers.

6. Install supports and trellises: If you're growing climbing or vining plants, add supports or trellises to your garden beds or containers to help with structural support and vertical growth. To support growing plants, use bamboo stakes, wire mesh, or wooden trellises. To avoid disturbing plant roots later on, place supports or trellises before planting.

7. Finishing Touches: After you've built your garden beds or containers, add finishing touches to improve their beauty and usefulness. Consider painting or staining wooden mattresses to improve durability and aesthetics. To help retain moisture, suppress weeds, and create a polished appearance, cover the surface of raised beds or containers with mulch or decorative stones.

8. Arrange and Plant: Place your garden beds or containers in the desired location, leaving enough space between each for access and airflow. Plant your vegetables, flowers, or herbs according to the recommended spacing and sunlight levels. After planting, properly water the plants and check soil moisture levels as they develop. Following these procedures and creating well-designed and constructed garden beds or containers will result in an attractive and productive garden environment that will thrive for many seasons. Whether you're gardening in a small urban location or a large backyard, the correct beds or containers may make the experience more fun and gratifying.

CHAPTER 5

Essential Tools and Equipment

Essential tools and equipment Gardening success requires that you have the proper tools and equipment. Having the right equipment on hand makes gardening upkeep easier and more effective, allowing you to enjoy your garden to its full potential.

Here's a list of important tools and equipment for any gardener:

1. Hand trowels are useful tools for planting, transplanting, and excavating small holes in the soil. For ease of use, choose a sturdy trowel with a comfortable grip.

2. A garden fork is excellent for turning soil, loosening compacted soil, and introducing soil additives. Choose a fork that has strong tines and a comfortable grip.

3. Pruning shears trim and shape plants, deadhead flowers, and prune tiny branches. Look for shears with sharp blades and ergonomic handles for a comfortable grip.

4. Garden Gloves: A pair of robust garden gloves will protect your hands from thorns, thorny plants, and rough surfaces. Choose gloves made of breathable, waterproof fabrics for the best comfort and protection.

5. Hand pruners, also known as secateurs, are useful for removing stems, branches, and tiny woody vegetation. Choose pruners with sharp bypass blades and a locking mechanism for further safety.

6. A garden rake is necessary for smoothing soil, spreading mulch, and clearing debris from planting areas. Choose a rake with strong ties and a comfortable grip for easy operation.

 7. Watering Can or Hose: To ensure that your plants receive enough moisture, irrigate your garden using a watering can or hose. For precision watering, use a sprinkler-equipped watering can or a hose with an adjustable nozzle.

8. A garden hoe cultivates soil, clears weeds, and makes furrows to put seeds in. Look for a hoe with a sharp blade and a long handle for ease of use.

9. Garden Knife: A garden knife is useful for cutting twine, opening soil or mulch bags, and doing other gardening activities. Choose a knife with a sharp, serrated blade and a comfortable grip.

10. A wheelbarrow or garden cart can easily transport large quantities of dirt, compost, or plants. Look for a durable, well-balanced model with pneumatic tires to provide smooth mobility over rough terrain.

11. Shovel: A sturdy shovel is required for digging planting holes, shifting dirt, and transporting mulch or compost. Choose a shovel with a sharp blade and a comfortable handle for long-term use.

12. A garden sprayer allows you to precisely apply fertilizers, insecticides, or herbicides to your plants. For maximum convenience, select a sprayer with adjustable nozzles and a comfortable pump handle.

13. Soil Test Kit: Use a soil test kit to determine the soil's pH, nutritional content, and texture. This invaluable tool contains critical information for soil preparation and amendment.

14. Knee Pads: A pair of cushioned knee pads or a kneeling pad will help protect your knees from strain and damage while kneeling or gardening for lengthy periods of time.

15. Pruning Saw: A pruning saw is excellent for cutting thicker branches, trimming thick stems, and shaping trees and plants. Select a saw with sharp, serrated teeth and a comfortable grip for effective cutting.

Investing in these basic tools and equipment will prepare you to tackle a variety of gardening activities while also maintaining a beautiful and healthy garden throughout the growing season. To achieve the greatest results, choose high-quality equipment that is sturdy, ergonomic, and tailored to your individual gardening demands.

Basic gardening tools are:

1. Hand Trowel: For planting, transplanting, and digging small holes in the soil, a hand trowel is required. It's ideal for working in confined spaces and loosening dirt around plants.

2. Pruning shears trim and shape plants, deadhead flowers, and prune tiny branches. They are essential for your garden's health and attractiveness.

3. Garden Gloves: A pair of robust garden gloves will protect your hands from thorns, thorny plants, and rough surfaces. They provide crucial hand protection when gardening.

4. A garden fork is a tool for turning soil, breaking up compacted dirt, and introducing soil additives. It's a useful tool for cultivating and aerating soil.

5. A garden rake is necessary for smoothing soil, spreading mulch, and clearing debris from planting areas. It helps to keep your garden beds nice and tidy.

6. Hand pruners, also known as secateurs, are useful for removing stems, branches, and tiny woody vegetation.

They are essential for precise trimming and deadheading.

7. Watering Can or Hose: To ensure that your plants receive enough moisture, irrigate your garden using a watering can or hose. Keep your plants watered, especially during the dry months.

8. Shovel: A robust shovel is required for digging planting holes, shifting dirt, and transporting mulch or compost. It's an essential tool for many gardening jobs.

9. Gardeners use a garden hoe to cultivate soil, clear weeds, and make furrows to put seeds in. It helps to keep your garden beds weed-free and aerated.

10. Garden Knife: A garden knife is useful for cutting twine, opening soil or mulch bags, and doing other gardening activities. It's a handy tool with several applications in the garden.

These fundamental gardening tools are vital for keeping your garden healthy and productive. With these tools in hand, you'll be ready to handle a variety of gardening jobs and keep your garden looking its best throughout the growing season.

Specialized Equipment

Specialized Equipment In addition to standard gardening tools, there are a few specialist pieces of equipment that may help you simplify various activities and improve your gardening experience. These specialist tools can greatly assist with specific gardening tasks.

Below are some examples of specialized gardening equipment:

1. Garden spades are heavy-duty digging tools with flat, squared-off blades. It's ideal for digging large planting holes, edging beds, and transporting heavy amounts of soil or compost. Garden spades are available in a variety of sizes and shapes to meet different gardening demands.

2. A garden fork with a D-handle is a heavy-duty instrument with sharp tines that is great for turning soil, breaking up compacted dirt, and introducing soil additives. The D-handle offers a comfortable grip and extra leverage for digging in difficult soil conditions.

3. A pruning saw with a telescoping handle is a useful instrument for cutting thicker branches, trimming thick stems, and shaping trees or plants. The telescopic handle allows you to prune high branches without the need for a ladder, making it safer and more effective.

4. An electric hedge trimmer is motorized equipment with reciprocating blades used to shape hedges, bushes, and topiaries. Electric hedge trimmers are lightweight, simple to operate, and offer accurate cutting action to produce clean, consistent cuts.

5. Soil Cultivator: A soil cultivator, also known as a rototiller or garden tiller, is a powered instrument with spinning tines used to break up soil, mix in fertilizers, and prep planting beds. Soil cultivators come in a variety of sizes and types, ranging from handheld devices for small gardens to bigger, self-propelled machines for larger areas.

6. Garden Sprayer with Adjustable Nozzle: A garden sprayer with an adjustable nozzle is used to precisely

administer fertilizers, insecticides, or herbicides to your garden. Adjustable nozzles allow you to tailor the spray pattern and intensity for a specific application.

7. A garden cart with a dumping function is a wheeled cart that can move large amounts of soil, compost, or plants throughout your garden. The dumping capability enables you to unload things with little effort, making gardening operations more efficient and less tiring.

8. A soil pH meter is a specialist gadget that measures the pH of your soil. It delivers quick feedback on soil acidity or alkalinity, allowing you to alter soil pH as needed to achieve the best growth conditions for your plants.

These specialized tools can help you do various gardening jobs more efficiently and successfully. Whether you're digging, trimming, tilling, or spraying, having the correct equipment makes gardening easier and more fun. Consider investing in specialist gardening equipment that aligns with your gardening goals and tastes.

Safety Precautions Gardening

Safety tips Gardening is a profitable and fun pastime, but it's important to emphasize safety to avoid accidents and injuries. Whether you're digging, trimming, or using chemicals, taking safety steps will help you have a successful and happy gardening experience.

Here are a few crucial safety things to remember:

1. Wear suitable attire and protective gear when gardening. Long trousers, strong closed-toe shoes, and work gloves can help prevent scratches, wounds, and bug bites. Wearing a wide-brimmed hat and sunscreen will help protect you from the sun's damaging rays, especially during peak hours.

2. Use garden tools. Properly: Follow the manufacturer's instructions and the intended function of your garden tools and equipment. Before using a tool, inspect it for damage or faults, and replace or repair any worn or damaged components. To minimize unintentional cuts or injuries when

using sharp equipment like pruners or saws, keep a firm hold and proceed with caution.

3. Lifting large goods, such as soil bags, pots, or plants, requires precise lifting techniques to minimize strain or damage. Bend your knees and raise your legs, keeping your back straight and your core muscles engaged for stability. Avoid twisting or jerking actions while lifting, and seek assistance if the thing is too large to lift alone.

4. Be mindful of animals: When gardening, be mindful of the possible threats provided by animals such as bees, wasps, spiders, and snakes. Take care not to damage nests or habitats, and use protective clothes if working in places where stinging or biting insects are present. If you come across wildlife, stay cool and gently back away to avoid eliciting a defensive response.

5. Handle Chemicals Safely: If you use pesticides, fertilizers, or other chemicals in your garden, use

them with caution and follow the label directions exactly. When working with chemicals, always wear protective gear, gloves, and glasses to avoid breathing fumes or putting products on your skin or eyes. Keep chemicals in their original containers in a safe place, out of reach of children and pets.

6. Watch Your Step: When gardening, keep your footing to prevent tripping or falling on uneven terrain, rocks, roots, or garden hoses. When walking on damp or slippery terrain, use handrails or assistance to navigate slopes or stairs. Keep paths free of waste and barriers to reduce the likelihood of accidents.

7. Stay Hydrated: Drink lots of water when gardening, especially if the weather is hot or you are doing heavy activities. Take regular rests in the shade to recover and cool down; avoid overexertion or working in high heat. Pay attention to symptoms of heat exhaustion or dehydration, such as dizziness,

weariness, or a fast heartbeat, and seek medical assistance if necessary.

8. When not in use, keep garden tools and equipment in a safe and orderly location to avoid accidents and injuries. Store sharp instruments, like pruners and saws, out of reach of children and pets in a designated area away from foot traffic. To prevent illegal access, store chemicals and insecticides in a secured cabinet or shed.

9. Know Your Limits: Understand your physical limitations and prevent overexertion when gardening. Pace yourself, and take pauses when necessary to rest and refuel. If you have a medical condition or mobility challenges, modify your gardening duties to meet your requirements or ask for help from family or friends.

11. Seek Professional Advice: If you're unclear about how to properly complete a gardening project or encounter a dangerous condition, consult a professional gardener, landscaper, or extension agency. If you are unable to do

a task safely on your own, do not be afraid to seek assistance or hire a professional.

Following these safety precautions may reduce the danger of accidents and injuries when gardening, ensuring a safe and pleasurable experience for yourself and others. Remember to be aware of your surroundings, use tools and equipment correctly, and take precautions to protect yourself from any risks. Gardening can be a safe and gratifying pastime for people of all ages and skill levels if they take the necessary measures and practice mindfulness.

Chapter 6

Starting with Seeds vs. Seedlings

When designing a garden, one of the first decisions you must make is whether to start your plants from seeds or buy seedlings from a nursery or garden shop. Both approaches have advantages and disadvantages, and the choice is based on criteria such as time, space, expertise, and personal taste.

Here's a contrast between beginning with seeds and seedlings: Starting with seeds:

1. **Variety Selection:** Starting with seeds provides a diverse range of plant alternatives, including heirloom varieties, uncommon species, and specialist cultivars that may not be accessible as seedlings. This allows you to experiment with numerous plant species and customize your garden to your unique needs and growth circumstances.

2. **Cost-effective:** Seeds are often less expensive than seedlings, especially if you plan to cultivate a large number of plants or varieties. A packet of seeds often contains many seeds, allowing you to grow a large

number of plants for a fraction of the cost of buying individual seedlings.

3. **Growing plants**: from seeds may be a fun and informative process, particularly for youngsters or inexperienced gardeners. It explains the plant lifecycle, from germination to maturity, and teaches useful skills like seed sowing, transplanting, and plant care.

4. **Timing Flexibility:** Starting with seeds allows us more flexibility in terms of timing and planting schedule. You may sow seeds indoors several weeks before the last frost date and move seedlings outside when the weather warms up, providing for a longer growth season for succession planting.

5. **Control over growth circumstances:** Starting with seeds gives you more control over the growth circumstances, such as soil quality, moisture levels, and temperature. This allows you to tailor the growing environment to your plants' individual demands, maximizing their development and output.

6. **Potential Difficulties:** Starting seeds requires careful attention to germination conditions such as temperature, moisture, and light levels. Some seeds may have low

germination rates or require special pre-treatment steps, such as stratification or scarification, complicating the procedure.

Firstly, start with seedlings:

1. Instant gratification: Purchasing seedlings allows you to transplant them into your garden and see results faster than beginning from seeds. This is especially tempting to gardeners who wish to enjoy their mature garden right away.

2. Starting with seedlings takes less time and effort than starting with seeds because the seedlings have already germinated and grown a root system. This might be useful for busy gardeners or people who have limited time for gardening tasks.

3. Seedlings are more durable and have a better success rate than seeds since they have already passed the sensitive germination period and are well-established. This lowers the chances of failure owing to reasons including inadequate germination, illness, or environmental stress.

4. Season Extension: Buying seedlings allows you to prolong the growing season by planting mature plants later or bringing them indoors for winter gardening. This is especially important for gardeners in areas with limited growth seasons or uncertain weather patterns.

5. Diversity Limitations: While seedlings are convenient and provide rapid results, they may have less diversity than growing from seeds. Nurseries and garden stores may have a variety of popular types, but they may not offer the same plant diversity as seeds.

6. Quality Considerations: To assure garden success, purchase healthy, disease-free seedlings from trustworthy providers. Before acquiring seedlings, carefully inspect them for symptoms of pests, illness, or stress, and avoid weak or damaged plants.

Understanding seeds and seedlings

Seeds are the first stage of a plant's life cycle, carrying all of the genetic information required for growth and development. Each seed is a little packet of promise that, given the correct conditions, may grow into a new plant. The size, shape, color, and texture of seeds vary greatly depending on the plant species to which they belong.

In flowering plants, pollen from the male reproductive organs (stamens) fertilizes the ovules within the female reproductive organs (pistils) to generate seeds. Once fertilized, the ovules grow into seeds, which are encased in protective seed coats that preserve the embryo and store nutrients until the conditions are right for germination. Germination is the process by which a seed sprouts and develops into a new plant.

It often involves water absorption, enzyme activation, and embryo enlargement when it emerges from dormancy and begins to develop into a seedling. Moisture, temperature, light, and oxygen levels all play a role in germination, which varies based on the plant type and seed properties.

Seedlings are young plants that have sprung from seeds and begun to develop above the soil surface.

As they settle into their new surroundings, they exhibit frail stems, immature leaves, and a weak root system. Seedlings grow and develop by absorbing nutrients and water from the surrounding soil, as well as stored energy within the seed. As seedlings grow, they go through a succession of developmental stages, including the appearance of genuine leaves, the formation of secondary roots, and the strengthening of stem components.

These phases are critical for developing a robust and healthy root system and preparing the seedling for later transplanting into the garden. Starting plants from seeds has various advantages, including a wider range of plant alternatives, lower costs, educational possibilities, and better control over growth conditions.

However, developing seeds into adult plants takes careful attention to germination requirements, patience, and time. Alternatively, buying seedlings delivers quick enjoyment and results, saving the time and effort necessary for gardening operations. Seedlings outperform seeds in terms of success rate and resilience, making them perfect for gardeners who wish to skip the germination stage and enjoy mature plants sooner.

Understanding the properties and life cycle of seeds and seedlings

Understanding the properties and life cycle of seeds and seedlings is critical to effective gardening. Knowing how seeds germinate, seedlings develop, and plants grow allows gardeners to make informed decisions regarding seed selection, planting procedures, and care practices to guarantee healthy and successful gardens.

Advantages and Disadvantages of Starting from Seeds

Pros and cons of starting with seeds Starting plants from seeds has a number of advantages and disadvantages, which should be considered when determining whether to start from seeds or seedlings.

The following are some of the primary advantages and disadvantages of starting with seeds:

Pros:

1. Variety: Starting from seeds gives you access to a diverse range of plant possibilities, including heirloom types, uncommon species, and specialist cultivars that may not be accessible as seedlings. This enables gardeners to experiment with numerous plant species and personalize their garden to their unique needs and growing circumstances.

2. Cost-effectiveness: Seeds are typically less expensive than seedlings, especially when cultivating a large number of plants or varieties. A single package of seeds often includes many seeds, allowing you to grow a large number of plants for a fraction of the cost of buying individual seedlings.

3. Growing plants from seeds may be a fun and informative process, particularly for youngsters or inexperienced gardeners. It explains the plant lifecycle, from germination to maturity, and teaches useful skills like seed sowing, transplanting, and plant care.

4. Timing Flexibility: Starting with seeds allows gardeners to be more flexible with their planting schedule. Start seeds indoors several weeks before the last frost date and transplant them outside when the weather warms to extend the growth season for succession planting.

5. Gardeners have more control over their growth circumstances when they start with seeds, such as soil quality, moisture levels, and temperature. This enables the tailoring of the growing environment to fit the plants' individual demands and enhance their development and output.

Cons:

1. Germination Challenges: Starting from seeds necessitates careful consideration of germination parameters such as temperature, moisture, and light levels. Some seeds may have low germination rates or require special pre-treatment steps, such as stratification or scarification, complicating the procedure.

2. Growing plants from seeds takes time and patience, since seeds must germinate, develop, and grow into mature plants

before they provide harvestable yields or flowers. This can be a longer process than purchasing seeds, taking weeks or even months of tending and care.

3. Seedlings that were started indoors may develop transplant shock when moved outside, especially if they have not been properly hardened off or have been exposed to extreme weather conditions. Transplant shock can limit growth and impair plant vitality, necessitating extra time and attention to recuperate.

4. Limited Availability: While seeds provide a diverse range of plant possibilities, some gardeners may discover that some specialist or hard-to-find types are not widely accessible as seeds. In such situations, purchasing seedlings may be the only way to access certain plant species.

5. Indoor Space: To start seeds indoors, you'll need enough space, light, and equipment, including seed trays, grow lights, and potting mix. Gardeners with little indoor space or poor illumination may struggle to properly start seeds indoors.

6. Greater chance of failure: Starting from seeds has a higher chance of failure than buying seedlings because seeds may

fail to germinate or succumb to pests, disease, or environmental stress. Gardeners must be prepared to diagnose and fix difficulties as they emerge in order to ensure effective germination and plant growth.

Individual tastes, gardening goals, and resources all influence whether to start with seeds or seedlings. While starting with seeds provides more diversity, cost-effectiveness, and instructional value, it also requires time, patience, and close attention to germination needs. In contrast, acquiring seedlings delivers rapid pleasure and outcomes, but may have limitations in terms of choice and availability.

Gardeners may make educated judgments about how to build flourishing and abundant gardens by assessing the benefits and drawbacks of each technique.

Pros and Cons of Using Seedlings

Using seedlings has advantages and disadvantages. Before deciding whether to start with seeds or seedlings, it is important to consider the various advantages and downsides of using seedlings in gardening.

Here are some of the key benefits and drawbacks of utilizing seedlings.

Pros:

1. Instant gratification: Purchasing seedlings allows you to transplant them into your garden and see results faster than beginning from seeds. This is especially tempting to gardeners who wish to enjoy their mature garden right away.

2. Seedlings take less time and effort to plant than seeds because they have already germinated and developed a root system. This might be useful for busy gardeners or people who have limited time for gardening tasks.

3. Seedlings are more durable and have a better success rate than seeds since they have already passed the sensitive germination period and are well-established. This lowers the

chances of failure owing to reasons including inadequate germination, illness, or environmental stress.

4. Season Extension: Seedlings allow you to prolong the growth period by planting mature plants later in the season or bringing them indoors for winter gardening. This is especially important for gardeners in areas with limited growth seasons or uncertain weather patterns.

5. Convenience: Purchasing seedlings from nurseries or garden stores saves time and effort compared to beginning seeds at home. Seedlings are available in a wide range of sizes and kinds, making it simple to locate plants that meet your garden's requirements and growth circumstances.

Cons:

1. Diversity Limitations: While seedlings are convenient and provide rapid results, they may have less diversity than growing from seeds. Nurseries and garden stores may have a variety of popular types, but they may not offer the same plant diversity as seeds.

2. Quality Considerations: To assure garden success, purchase healthy, disease-free seedlings from trustworthy

providers. Before acquiring seedlings, carefully inspect them for symptoms of pests, illness, or stress, and avoid weak or damaged plants.

3. Cost: Seedlings might be more expensive than seeds, especially if you're growing a big garden with numerous types. While seedlings may be more expensive at first, the higher success rate and reduced time and effort required for gardening duties may make the investment worthwhile for certain gardeners.

4. Transferring seedlings from their original containers to garden soil may cause transplant shock, especially if they have not been adequately hardened off or have been exposed to extreme weather conditions. Transplant shock can limit growth and impair plant vitality, necessitating extra time and attention to recuperate.

5. Dependence on Suppliers: If supplies are scarce or unavailable, depending on nurseries or garden centers for seedlings may limit your ability to obtain plants. To assure availability and selection, prepare ahead of time and buy seedlings early in the season. Individual tastes, gardening

goals, and resources all influence whether to utilize seedlings or start from seeds.

While seedlings offer ease, fast results, and a higher success rate, there may be limitations in terms of variety, quality, and cost. Gardeners may make educated judgments about how to build flourishing and abundant gardens by assessing the benefits and drawbacks of each technique.

Seed-Starting Techniques

Seed-starting procedures include a number of ways for germinating seeds and raising seedlings until they are suitable for transplantation into the garden.

These strategies seek to produce ideal circumstances for seed germination, seedling development, and general plant health.

Here are some typical seed-starting methods:

1. Indoor Seed Starting: Indoor seed beginning is planting seeds indoors, usually in trays or pots filled with seed-starting mix or potting soil. Seeds are planted at the proper depth and spacing, softly covered with soil, and gently watered to maintain enough hydration. Seed trays are put in a warm, well-lit environment, such as a sunny windowsill or under grow lights, to promote germination and seedling growth. Proper ventilation and air movement are essential for preventing damping-off disease and promoting healthy seedling growth. As seedlings mature, they may require thinning or transfer to bigger pots to avoid overpopulation and resource competition.

2. Direct Sowing: Direct sowing includes putting seeds directly into garden soil or outdoor containers, eliminating the need for indoor seeding. Seeds are planted at the proper depth and spacing in prepared garden beds or containers, taking into account soil temperature, moisture, and sunshine needs. Direct sowing is appropriate for seeds of hardy plants that can withstand outside conditions, such as vegetables, herbs, and annual flowers. The success of direct sowing is dependent on soil preparation, meteorological conditions, and pest management.

3. Germination Techniques: A variety of germination procedures may be employed to increase seed germination rates and accelerate the process. Scarification is the process of nicking or scratching the seed coat to improve water absorption and seedling emergence, especially for hard-coated seeds. Stratification includes exposing seeds to cold, damp temperatures in order to break dormancy and replicate winter conditions. This is a typical name for the seeds of perennial plants native to colder areas. Soaking seeds in water or a diluted hydrogen peroxide solution will soften the seed coverings and promote germination.

4. Bottom Watering: Bottom watering is a seed-starting method that includes watering seed trays or containers from the bottom rather than the top. Seed trays are placed in a shallow tray or bigger container full of water, allowing the soil to absorb moisture from the bottom by capillary action. Bottom watering prevents soil disturbance and lowers the danger of damping-off disease by keeping the soil surface dry. It also promotes downward growth and reduces the risk of soggy soil.

5. Harden off seedlings: Harden off seedlings before transferring them outside to progressively adjust them to the outside environment. Begin by exposing seedlings to outside circumstances for brief periods of time every day, progressively increasing the duration and intensity of exposure over 1-2 weeks.

To avoid stress and injury, protect seedlings from direct sunlight, wind, and temperature extremes throughout the hardening off phase. Once seedlings have fully adapted, they may be transferred into garden soil or outdoor pots with little chance of transplant shock.

These seed-starting methods can be modified and combined to meet the individual requirements of various plant species and growth conditions. By may effectively start seeds and produce healthy, robust seedlings for transplanting into their gardens by following appropriate practices and providing ideal growth conditions.

Planting Your Garden

Planting your garden is a fun and gratifying process that requires carefully selecting and arranging plants in the right spots to create a beautiful and practical outdoor environment. Whether you're starting with seeds, seedlings, or established plants, appropriate planting procedures are critical to the success and vitality of your garden.

Here's a complete guide to planting your garden:

 1. Site Selection: Determine the best site for your garden based on characteristics including sunshine exposure, soil quality, drainage, and closeness to water supplies. Consider the individual demands of the plants you wish to cultivate and choose a location with adequate sunshine, moisture, and soil type.

 2. Soil preparation: Involves loosening the soil using a garden fork or tiller to promote drainage and aeration. Remove any weeds, rocks, or debris from the planting area, and add organic matter like compost, aged manure, or peat moss to boost fertility and improve soil structure.

3. Plant Selection: Choose plants that are appropriate for your climate, growth circumstances, and garden design choices. When selecting plants for your garden, consider plant size, growth habits, bloom duration, color, and texture. Pay attention to plant labels or consult gardening guides to ensure optimum spacing and compatibility among plant varieties.

4. Planting Technique: Dig holes that are somewhat broader and deeper than the plant's root ball or container. Gently take the plant from its container, plucking out any roots that are root-bound, and set it in the center of the planting hole at the same level it was growing in the container. Backfill the hole with dirt, carefully firming it around the roots to remove air pockets.

5. Watering: Water newly planted plants vigorously right away to settle the soil and provide optimal root-to-soil contact. Water the soil on a regular basis during the establishment stage to keep it wet but not saturated. Use a watering can or hose with a gentle spray nozzle to distribute water to the plant's base while avoiding soaking the leaves.

6. Mulching: To conserve moisture, control weeds, and regulate soil temperature, cover newly planted plants with an organic mulch such as shredded bark, wood chips, or straw. Leave a tiny space between the mulch and the plant stem to minimize moisture-related problems like decay or illness. Replenish mulch as required to provide a continuous covering throughout the growth season.

7. To ensure healthy development and establishment, fertilize newly planted plants using a balanced, slow-release fertilizer. Follow the application rate and time directions on the label, and avoid over-fertilizing, which can lead to nutritional imbalances or root burn. Consider utilizing organic fertilizers or soil amendments to promote long-term soil health and sustainability.

8. Maintenance: Keep an eye out for symptoms of stress, insect infestation, or disease in newly planted plants, and respond quickly to any problems that occur. Support tall or vining plants using pegs or trellises to prevent lodging or damage from wind or heavy rain. Prune or deadhead plants as needed to keep them in shape, promote blooming, and remove wasted flowers.

9. Monitoring and Care: On a regular basis, check your garden for signs of growth, flowering, or fruiting, and modify your watering, fertilizing, and pest control techniques as needed. Keep a watch out for indicators of nutrient deficiency, water stress, or insect damage, and take proactive steps to keep your plants healthy and vibrant. Enjoy the beauty and richness of your garden as it develops and changes over time.

To build a growing and lively outdoor environment, carefully design your garden, pay attention to detail, and maintain it on a regular basis. By using appropriate planting techniques and providing ideal growth conditions, you may create a beautiful and fruitful garden that will offer delight and satisfaction for years to come.

Timing Your Planting

Planting at the right time is critical to the success of your garden, as well as increasing plant growth and output. Climate, weather patterns, soil temperature, and the special demands of each plant species are all considered while planting at the appropriate time.

Here's a full breakdown of when to plant:

1. Frost Dates: Determine the average date of the final spring and first fall frosts in your area. These frost dates are key milestones for organizing your planting schedule and choosing frost-tolerant or cold-hardy plants. Use local gardening resources or internet tools to discover frost date projections for your area.

2. Early Spring Planting: Begin planting cool-season vegetables like peas, lettuce, spinach, carrots, and radishes as soon as the soil is workable in early spring. These crops can withstand lower temperatures and be planted several weeks before the last frost date. To guarantee ideal germination and development conditions, monitor soil temperature and moisture levels.

3. Late Spring Planting: Plant warm-season crops like tomatoes, peppers, cucumbers, squash, and beans after the last frost has passed. These crops require warm soil and air conditions for growth and should be planted after the threat of frost has passed. To progressively adapt seedlings to outdoor settings, start them indoors and harden them off before transplanting them outside.

4. Summer Planting: After soil temperatures have warmed up enough, plant heat-loving crops including maize, melons, eggplant, and okra in late spring to early summer. These crops thrive in hot weather and require full sunlight and appropriate moisture to produce a large harvest. To avoid stress and wilting, keep soil moisture levels under control and provide additional watering during dry spells.

5. Fall Planting: For a fall harvest, plant cool-season crops in late summer or early fall to extend the growing season. Leafy greens, root vegetables, brassicas, and herbs are examples of crops that can withstand lower temperatures and fewer daylight hours. Planting these crops in late July allows them to develop before the first fall frost, resulting in fresh produce far into the autumn.

6. Succession Planting: To increase your garden's yield and lengthen the harvest season, use succession planting. Planting fresh crops in the same location after previous harvests allows you to maximize available growing space and stagger planting dates. Plan your succession planting program around crop maturity dates and seasonal weather trends.

7. Weather Considerations: When planning your planting schedule, keep in mind weather forecasts and seasonal trends. Avoid planting during periods of excessive heat, cold, or heavy rain, since these circumstances can stress plants and impair their growth and development. Plant on cloudy days, early morning or late afternoon, to reduce transplant shock and water stress.

8. Soil Temperature: To ensure that seeds germinate and plants grow properly, keep track of soil temperature. Use a soil thermometer to determine the soil temperature at planting depth, and follow the temperature requirements for each plant species. Warm-season crops typically require soil temperatures of at least 60°F (15°C) to germinate, but cool-season crops may withstand lower temperatures.

9. Microclimates: In your garden, make use of microclimates to produce ideal growth conditions for various plants. South-facing slopes, protected spots, or sites near buildings or walls may have somewhat higher temperatures and longer growing seasons, allowing you to plant heat-loving crops or fragile perennials that would not survive elsewhere in your garden.

10. Gardening Calendar: Throughout the growing season, use a gardening calendar or notebook to record planting dates, weather conditions, and crop performance. Keep track of your planting successes and failures, as well as any changes or improvements to your planting schedule or procedures. In the coming seasons, a gardening calendar can help you plan and arrange your garden more successfully. Timing your planting requires careful consideration of elements such as frost dates, weather conditions, soil temperature, and your plants' individual requirements.

Planting Techniques for Optimal Growth

Proper planting techniques are essential for growing healthy, thriving plants in your garden. Whether you're planting seeds, seedlings, or mature plants, proper planting techniques can help promote strong root development, reduce transplant shock, and optimize growing conditions for your plants.

Here's a detailed overview of appropriate planting techniques:

1. Site Selection: Determine the best location for your plants based on factors such as sunlight exposure, soil quality, drainage, and spacing requirements. Consider the specific requirements of the plants you're planting, and choose a location that offers the best growing conditions for optimal growth and performance.

2. Soil Preparation: To improve drainage and aeration, loosen the soil with a garden fork or tiller before planting. Remove any weeds, rocks, or debris from the planting area, and add organic matter like compost, aged manure, or peat moss to boost fertility and improve soil structure.

3. Digging Planting Holes: Create planting holes that are slightly wider and deeper than the plant's root ball or container. For seeds, dig a planting furrow or individual holes spaced according to the recommended planting distance for each crop. Make sure the planting holes are well-spaced to allow for proper root development and airflow between plants.

4. Planting Depth: Plant seeds and seedlings at the appropriate depth for their specific needs. Plant seeds at a depth two to three times their diameter to ensure good soil-to-seed contact and germination. Plant seedlings and transplants at the same depth as they were in their containers, with the top of the root ball level with the soil surface.

5. Handling Seedlings: Gently remove seedlings from their containers by squeezing or tapping the sides to loosen the roots. Avoid pulling or yanking on the stems, as this can cause damage to delicate roots or stems. If the seedlings are root-bound, gently tease out the roots to promote outward growth and prevent circling.

6. Backfilling: Place the plant or seedling in the center of the planting hole and fill it with soil, firming it gently around the roots to remove air pockets. Check that the plant is stable and upright in the soil, with no exposed roots or gaps near the root ball. To help settle the soil and promote root growth, thoroughly water the newly planted plant.

7. Watering: To ensure adequate moisture and root-to-soil contact, water newly planted plants right away. Deep, thorough watering will penetrate the root zone and encourage roots to establish themselves in the surrounding soil. Water frequently during the establishment period to keep the soil evenly moist but not waterlogged, especially in hot or dry weather.

8. Mulching: To conserve moisture, suppress weeds, and regulate soil temperature, cover newly planted plants with an organic mulch such as shredded bark, wood chips, or straw. Leave a tiny space between the mulch and the plant stem to minimize moisture-related problems like decay or illness. Replenish mulch as required to provide a continuous covering throughout the growth season.

9. Staking and Support: For tall or vining plants, use stakes, trellises, or cages to prevent lodging or damage from wind or heavy rain. Install stakes or supports at the time of planting or soon after to avoid disturbing the roots once the plants have established themselves. To prevent stem damage or growth restriction, tie plants to supports with soft twine or plant ties.

10. Maintenance: Keep an eye out for symptoms of stress, insect infestation, or disease in newly planted plants, and respond quickly to any problems that occur. Provide additional support, pruning, or training as needed to keep the plant in shape and promote healthy growth.

Water, fertilize, and mulch plants on a regular basis to promote vigor and productivity during the growing season. Using proper planting techniques, you can grow healthy and resilient plants in your garden and create a beautiful and thriving outdoor space. Pay attention to site selection, soil preparation, planting depth, watering, and maintenance practices to ensure your garden's success and enjoy a bountiful harvest or vibrant landscape for many years.

Space and Depth Guidelines

Spacing and depth guidelines are critical when planting seeds, seedlings, or transplants in your garden. Proper spacing ensures that plants have enough room to grow, have access to sunlight and airflow, and make the best use of the available space. Depth guidelines help seeds develop and germinate properly, as well as establish healthy root systems for transplants.

Here's a detailed overview of plant spacing and depth guidelines:

Spacing Guidelines:

1. Read the planting instructions: For specific spacing recommendations for each plant species, consult seed packets, plant tags, or gardening books. Spacing requirements vary according to plant size, growth habit, and mature plant dimensions.

2. Plant-to-Plant Spacing: To avoid overcrowding and resource competition, space plants based on their mature size and growth habits. Follow plant-to-plant spacing guidelines to ensure proper airflow, sunlight penetration, and access to nutrients and water.

3. Row Spacing: For row planting, space rows apart based on the plant's needs and available growing space. Allow enough space between rows for walking, weeding, and maintenance tasks, taking into account the size of garden tools and equipment.

4. Square Foot Gardening: In intensive gardening methods like square foot gardening, plants are spaced closer together to maximize space and productivity. To achieve the best plant density and yield, adhere to the square-foot gardening spacing guidelines.

5. Companion Planting: To maximize space while improving plant health and productivity, use companion planting techniques. Plant compatible species together to make the best use of available space, discourage pests, and improve soil fertility through mutually beneficial interactions.

Depth Guidelines:

1. **Read the seed packet instructions:** When planting seeds, please refer to the seed packet instructions for specific depth requirements. Seed depth varies depending on the size and type of seed, as well as each plant species' germination requirements.

2. **Plant seeds at the recommended depth** to ensure successful germination and seedling emergence. In general, plant seeds at a depth two to three times their diameter, with larger seeds planted deeper.

3. **Transplant Depth:** When planting seedlings or transplants, keep them at the same level they were growing in their containers. Make sure the top of the root ball is level with the soil surface to avoid burying the stem or exposing the roots.

4. **Root Depth:** When determining planting depth, keep in mind the plants' root depth requirements. Shallow-rooted plants, such as lettuce or radishes, need shallower planting depths, whereas deep-rooted plants, such as tomatoes or

peppers, may require deeper planting to establish a strong root system.

5. Soil Texture and Moisture: When determining planting depth, take into account soil texture and moisture levels. Plant seeds or transplants in well-drained soil to avoid waterlogging and encourage healthy root growth. To ensure optimal growing conditions, adjust planting depth accordingly based on soil moisture and texture. When planting your garden, follow spacing and depth guidelines to optimize plant growth, maximize space utilization, and create healthy and productive crops or landscapes. To ensure your garden's success, follow specific recommendations for each plant species and adjust spacing and depth based on growing conditions and gardening practices.

Watering a newly planted garden

Watering newly planted gardens is critical for plant establishment and growth. Proper watering techniques help plants establish strong root systems, avoid transplant shock, and improve overall plant health and vigor.

Here's a detailed guide to watering newly planted gardens:

1. Watering Frequency: Newly planted gardens require regular watering to keep the soil evenly moist but not overly wet. Water plants deeply immediately after planting to ensure proper root establishment. Afterward, monitor soil moisture levels on a regular basis and provide water as needed, especially during hot or dry weather.

2. Water newly planted gardens: Early in the morning or late in the afternoon to limit evaporation and reduce the risk of fungal infections. Avoid watering during the hottest part of the day because water droplets on foliage can act as magnifying glasses, causing sunburn or scorching of the leaves.

3. **Deep Watering:** To promote deep root development and avoid shallow root systems, water deeply and thoroughly. Apply water to the root zone slowly and evenly, allowing moisture to permeate the entire root system. Water the soil deeply enough to moisten it up to the plant's root system depth, which is typically 6 to 12 inches.

4. Watering Technique: Use a watering can, hose with a gentle spray nozzle, or drip irrigation system to deliver water directly to the plant's base. Water at a moderate, constant rate to allow water to infiltrate the soil and prevent runoff. Aim to moisten the whole root zone while avoiding soil compaction and erosion.

5. Mulching: To conserve moisture, suppress weeds, and regulate soil temperature, cover newly planted plants with an organic mulch, such as shredded bark, wood chips, or straw. Mulch reduces evaporation and prevents the soil surface from drying out between watering, helping to retain soil moisture.

6. Soil Moisture Monitoring: Insert your finger into the soil around the plant's base on a regular basis to check for moisture levels. If the soil is dry to the touch, it is time to water. Avoid overwatering, which can result in soggy soil, root rot, and other moisture-related problems. Adjust watering frequency and volume based on weather, plant requirements, and soil moisture levels.

7. Drought Stress: Look for signs of drought stress, such as wilting, yellowing, or curling leaves, and adjust your watering schedule accordingly. During prolonged droughts or extreme heat, plants may require more frequent watering to maintain adequate moisture levels and avoid dehydration.

8. Watering newly transplanted seedlings or plants is especially important for reducing transplant shock and promoting quick root development. Water transplants immediately after planting, and continue to water them regularly until they show indications of new growth and adjust to their new surroundings.

9. To avoid water stress, keep soil moisture levels steady throughout the growth season. Allowing soil to dry fully between watering can stress plants and slow their development and output. During dry spells or periods of insufficient rainfall, provide supplemental irrigation to ensure that plants receive adequate moisture.

CHAPTER 7

Garden Care

Caring for your garden is an ongoing process that requires regular maintenance, monitoring, and attention to your plants' needs. By giving your garden the proper care and attention, you can promote healthy growth, prevent pests and diseases, and maximize its beauty and productivity.

Here's a detailed overview of garden maintenance:

Soil Health: To maintain soil fertility and structure, add organic matter like compost, aged manure, or mulch. To ensure that your plants grow optimally, test the soil pH and nutrient levels on a regular basis. Crop rotation and cover cropping can help prevent soil depletion and reduce the risk of pests and diseases. Monitor soil moisture levels and provide supplemental irrigation as needed to avoid drought stress and promote healthy plant growth.

Watering: To promote deep root growth and avoid shallow root systems, water plants deeply and infrequently. Water early in the morning or late in the afternoon to maintain consistent moisture levels and reduce evaporation. Regularly monitor soil moisture levels and adjust watering frequency and volume to suit weather conditions and plant requirements. Mulch can help retain soil moisture, suppress weeds, and regulate soil temperature, reducing the need for frequent watering.

Weeding: To avoid competition for water, nutrients, and sunlight, remove weeds from your garden on a regular basis. Mulch helps suppress weed growth and makes it easier to pull weeds when they emerge. Hand-pull weeds or use a hoe or cultivator to remove them from the soil surface, taking care not to harm nearby plants. To prevent weeds from becoming overwhelming and spreading throughout the garden, be vigilant and address them as soon as possible.

Pest and Disease Management: Regularly check plants for signs of pest infestation or disease, such as wilting, yellowing, or distorted growth. Identify pests and diseases precisely in order to determine the most effective control methods, such as cultural, mechanical, biological, or chemical controls. Use integrated pest management (IPM) techniques to reduce the use of chemical pesticides and promote ecological balance in your garden. Encourage beneficial insects, birds, and other natural predators to control pest populations and reduce the need for chemical treatments.

Pruning and Training: Regular pruning helps to remove dead or diseased branches, improve airflow and light penetration, and shape plant growth. Use sharp, clean pruning tools to make precise cuts while minimizing plant damage. To maximize space utilization, train vining or sprawling plants like tomatoes, cucumbers, and grapes to grow on trellises, stakes, or cages. Pruning fruit trees and shrubs promotes fruit production, improves tree health, and keeps them manageable in size and shape.

Fertilizing: Fertilize your plants on a regular basis with balanced, slow-release fertilizers to ensure healthy growth and productivity. Follow the recommended application rates and timing for each plant species, taking into account soil fertility, plant requirements, and seasonal growth cycles. Consider using organic fertilizers or soil amendments to improve soil health, promote microbial activity, and increase nutrient availability for plants. Avoid over fertilization, which can cause nutrient imbalances, fertilizer burns, and environmental pollution.

Harvesting and maintenance: Harvest fruits, vegetables, herbs, and flowers on a regular basis to promote long-term growth and prevent over-ripening or seed formation. Remove spent blooms and deadhead flowers, and trim back overgrown or leggy growth to promote new growth and extend flowering. To ensure optimal performance and longevity, clean and maintain garden tools and equipment on a regular basis. To maintain organization, keep records of planting dates, varieties, and garden tasks to track progress and plan future planting and maintenance activities.

Watering

Watering is an essential component of garden care that has a direct impact on the health and growth of your plants. Proper watering techniques ensure that plants get the moisture they need to thrive while reducing water waste and potential problems like root rot or disease.

Here's a detailed review of watering practices:

1. Watering frequency varies according to plant species, soil type, weather conditions, and stage of growth. In general, it is better to water deeply and infrequently than shallowly and frequently. Allow the soil to dry slightly between watering's to promote deep root growth and avoid waterlogged conditions.

2. Water plants early in the morning or late in the afternoon to avoid evaporative water loss and the danger of fungal infections. Avoid watering during the warmest part of the day because water droplets on foliage can function as magnifying glasses, causing sunburn or blistering of the leaves.

3. Soil Moisture: Regularly check the moisture content of the soil using your finger or a soil moisture meter. When the top inch or two of soil is dry to the touch, water it. To guarantee ideal growth circumstances, adjust the frequency and volume of watering according to the weather, plant demands, and soil moisture.

4. Watering Technique: Use a watering can, hose with a gentle spray nozzle, or drip irrigation system to send water

straight to the plant's base. Water slowly and steadily so that water may enter the soil and reach the root zone. Whenever possible, avoid overhead watering because it promotes fungal infections and wastes water.

5. Deep Watering: To promote root development and drought resistance, water deeply and thoroughly. Apply water gently and evenly to the root zone, allowing moisture to permeate the whole root system. Water thoroughly enough to wet the soil up to the plant's root system depth, which is usually 6 to 12 inches.

6. Mulching: To conserve moisture, control weeds, and regulate soil temperature, cover plants with an organic mulch such as shredded bark, wood chips, or straw. Mulch helps to maintain soil moisture by minimizing evaporation and preventing the soil surface from drying out between watering.

7. Container plants require more water than ground plants because they dry up more quickly. Check the moisture levels in the container daily and add water as needed to keep the soil equally wet but not saturated. Consider utilizing self-

watering containers or adding water-retaining chemicals to potting mixes to help preserve moisture.

8. Drought Stress: Look for signs of drought stress, such as wilting, yellowing, or curled leaves, and adjust your watering schedule accordingly. During extended droughts or excessive heat, plants may require more frequent watering to maintain proper moisture levels and avoid dehydration. Consider installing a rain gauge or moisture sensor to monitor soil moisture levels and guide watering decisions.

9. Maintaining regular soil moisture levels throughout the growing season promotes healthy plant development and production. Allowing the soil to completely dry between watering can stress plants and impede their development and productivity. During dry spells or periods of inadequate rainfall, use supplemental irrigation to ensure that plants receive appropriate moisture.

Following the correct watering procedures can help your garden survive and develop throughout the growing season. To guarantee your plants' health and vitality, pay attention to their demands, soil moisture levels, and ambient conditions, and adapt your watering habits accordingly.

Weeding

Weeding is a necessary chore in garden management that entails eliminating undesired plants, or weeds, from your garden beds or growing regions. Weeds compete with attractive plants for nutrients, water, and sunshine, and if not controlled, they may swiftly overtake a garden.

Here's a full explanation of weeding techniques:

1. Regular Inspection: Keep an eye out for weed development in your garden beds or growing regions. Walk around your garden multiple times every week, especially during the growing season, to locate and remove weeds before they become entrenched and spread.

2. Hand pulling is the most popular and effective way to remove weeds from garden beds. Wear gloves to protect your hands, and use a kneeling pad or cushion to make the process easier. Grab weeds firmly around the base, as close to the soil surface as possible, then gently pull them upward to remove the entire plant, including the roots.

3. Weed Tools: Use a hand weedier, garden trowel, or hoe to help remove bigger or more persistent weeds. Insert the instrument into the soil near the weed's base, and pry or slice beneath the root system to loosen and remove the plant. Choose tools that are suitable for the size and density of the weeds in your garden.

4. To keep weeds from establishing and spreading throughout your garden, weed early and regularly. Remove weeds when they are young and actively developing, before they blossom and set seed. Regular, consistent weeding is critical for controlling weed populations and preventing future weed problems.

5. Mulching: Apply a layer of organic mulch, such as shredded bark, wood chips, or straw, around plants to discourage weed development and make it easier to uproot weeds when they appear. Mulch helps to smother weeds by limiting sunlight and keeping weed seeds from developing. Replenish mulch as required to provide a continuous covering throughout the growth season.

6. Weed Prevention: Take proactive measures to prevent weed development in your garden beds. Minimize soil disturbance to prevent buried weed seeds from germinating.

Consider placing landscaping fabric or cardboard under mulch as a weed barrier, especially in weed-prone regions.

7. Weed Management: Regularly monitor weed populations and respond promptly to any weed problems that arise. Maintain vigilance and eliminate weeds before they spread and compete with valuable plants for resources. Consider employing organic pesticides or weed suppressants as part of a comprehensive weed control plan.

8. Persistent Weeds: Certain weeds may be more difficult to control and require additional efforts to remove. Persistent weeds with deep taproots or extensive rhizomes may require repeated manual plucking or targeted pesticide treatments to prevent regrowth. For information on how to manage specific weed species, consult your local gardening resources or extension services.

9. Weed Disposal: Properly dispose of weeds to keep them from re-growing in your garden or spreading to other places. Pull weeds and place them in a designated compost pile or green trash container, making sure they are entirely dead and unable to regenerate. To keep weed seeds from sprouting in your compost, avoid composting mature weeds. By incorporating regular weeding into your garden management regimen, you can keep weed populations under control while also creating a healthy, thriving garden environment for your plants. Maintain a proactive, attentive, and thorough approach to weed management, and you will be able to appreciate the beauty and productivity of your garden without the intrusion of undesired weeds.

Fertilization

Fertilizing is an important part of garden maintenance since it provides plants with the necessary nutrients to support healthy growth, vitality, and output. Fertilizers boost the soil's inherent nutritional content, ensuring that plants have access to the nutrients they require for proper growth and development.

Here is a full summary of fertilization practices:

1. Soil Testing: Begin by testing your soil to determine its nutrient content and pH balance. Soil testing provides essential information regarding nutrient deficits or imbalances, allowing you to adjust your fertilization

program to your plants' exact requirements. Collect soil samples from various sections of your garden and submit them to a reliable soil testing facility for examination.

2. Choose the Right Fertilizer: Choose a fertilizer formulation that corresponds to your plants' nutritional requirements, as well as the recommendations based on your soil tests. These three numbers on fertilizer labels signify the amount of nitrogen (N), phosphorus (P), and potassium (K) in their composition. For general-purpose applications, use a balanced fertilizer (e.g., 10-10-10) or pick specialist fertilizers tailored to specific plant needs.

3. Application Rates: Use the suggested application rates for the type of fertilizer, plant species, and stage of growth. Over-fertilization can cause nutritional imbalances, fertilizer burn, and environmental contamination, whereas under-fertilization can result in nutrient shortages and poor plant development. Use a calibrated spreader or measuring cup to distribute fertilizer evenly and precisely.

4. Timing: Fertilizer should be applied at the proper times during the growing season to promote plant growth. Fertilize plants in early spring to stimulate rapid development, then

again in late spring or early summer to maintain growth throughout the growing season. Avoid fertilizing plants under drought or heat stress, as it may worsen plant stress and limit fertilizer efficacy.

5. Fertilizer can be applied in a variety of ways, such as broadcasting, side dressing, foliar spraying, or soil soaking. Spread granular fertilizers uniformly over the soil's surface and thoroughly water to ensure that nutrients reach the root zone. Side-dress plants by spreading fertilizer in a thin band along the plant's root zone, avoiding direct contact with stems or leaves. To supply nutrients directly to plant leaves or roots, apply liquid fertilizers through foliar sprays or soil drenches.

6. Organic Fertilizers: Organic fertilizers or soil amendments can help improve soil health, encourage microbial activity, and increase nutrient availability for plants. Compost, aged manure, fish emulsion, and seaweed extract are examples of organic fertilizers that give slow-release nutrients while also improving soil structure. To improve plant nutrition and soil fertility, incorporate organic matter into the soil or use it as a top dressing.

7. Specialist fertilizers: Use specialist fertilizers or additives to correct nutritional deficits or improve plant performance. Products like bone meal, blood meal, kelp meal, and Epsom salt supply targeted nutrients that may be deficient in your soil or required by certain plant species. When using specialized fertilizers, always follow the package recommendations to avoid over-application or nutritional imbalances.

8. Watering after Fertilizing: After fertilizing, water the plants thoroughly to dissolve the nutrients and distribute them equally throughout the root zone. Irrigate plants right after you apply fertilizer to avoid fertilizer burn and ensure that nutrients are quickly available to plants. Avoid adding fertilizer to dry soil because salts can collect and harm plant roots.

9. Maintenance: Keep track of plant growth and reaction to fertilizer, and alter your fertilization schedule as needed depending on plant requirements and soil test findings. Avoid excessive fertilization, which can cause nutrient runoff, groundwater pollution, and environmental damage. Use appropriate fertilizer techniques to encourage healthy

plant development while reducing environmental effects. By following the correct fertilization procedures, you can supply your plants with the nutrients they require to live and flourish throughout the growing season. Pay attention to soil conditions, plant demands, and environmental circumstances, and adapt your fertilizer schedule accordingly to guarantee your garden's health and vitality.

Mulching

Mulching is a useful garden care strategy that involves adding a layer of organic or inorganic material to the soil surface around plants. Mulch has several functions, including retaining soil moisture, inhibiting weed development, controlling soil temperature, and promoting soil health.

Here's a full review of mulching techniques:

1. Mulch Materials: There are several types of mulch materials available, both organic and inorganic. Organic mulches like shredded bark, wood chips, straw, compost, leaves, and grass clippings degrade over time, contributing

organic matter to the soil and strengthening its structure. Inorganic mulches, such as plastic sheeting, landscaping fabric, or gravel, provide long-term weed control and moisture retention but do not provide organic matter to the soil.

2. To achieve excellent weed control and moisture retention, apply mulch to a depth of 2 to 4 inches around plants. Thicker layers of mulch may cause excessive moisture retention and soil compaction, whereas thinner layers may provide insufficient weed control or moisture conservation. Maintain a continuous layer of mulch throughout the growth season, refilling as necessary.

3. Mulch reduces weed development by blocking sunlight and preventing weed seeds from developing. Mulch around plants and between rows will act as a weed barrier, reducing the need for hand weeding. Before spreading mulch, make sure the soil surface is free of weeds to prevent them from sprouting through the mulch layer.

4. Soil Moisture Conservation: Mulch functions as a protective barrier, limiting evaporation from the soil surface. Apply mulch uniformly around plants to create a moisture-

retaining layer that reduces water loss and helps to maintain stable soil moisture levels. To encourage deep root development and maximize the benefits of mulch, water plants deeply and infrequently.

5. Mulch insulates the soil and helps to maintain its temperature by acting as a buffer against severe heat or cold. Mulch keeps the soil cool in hot weather and minimizes temperature changes that might cause plant stress. In cold weather, mulch works as insulation, shielding plant roots from freezing temperatures and frost damage.

6. Soil Health: Organic mulches decay over time, contributing organic matter to the soil while enhancing fertility, structure, and microbial activity. Organic mulches decompose and release nutrients into the soil, providing a natural source of plant sustenance. Incorporate mulch into the soil on a regular basis to improve soil health and promote long-term sustainability.

7. Application Techniques: Apply mulch gently around the base of plants, allowing a little space between the mulch and the plant stem to minimize moisture-related difficulties like rot or disease. Spread mulch uniformly throughout the soil

surface, taking care not to pile it up against tree trunks or plant stems, which can provide ideal conditions for pests and diseases.

8. Mulch Maintenance: Check the mulch on a regular basis and refill it as needed to provide a constant covering throughout the growth season. Rake mulch on a regular basis to fluff it up and avoid compaction, which can hinder ventilation and water penetration. Remove any weeds or debris that may have accumulated on the mulch surface to keep it looking clean and pleasant. Mulching can help to enhance soil health, preserve moisture, reduce weeds, and create an environment that promotes plant development and production. Choose mulch materials that are suitable for your garden's needs and tastes, and then apply mulch appropriately to maximize its benefits while also improving the appearance and sustainability of your garden.

Pest and Disease Management

Pest and disease management is a critical component of garden care that entails recognizing, preventing, and managing pests and diseases in order to protect plants from damage and maintain their health and production. Gardeners may reduce their dependency on chemical pesticides by employing integrated pest management (IPM) strategies that maintain ecological balance in the garden.

Here's a full summary of pest and disease management practices:

1. Pest Identification: Inspect plants on a regular basis for symptoms of pest infestation, such as chewed leaves, holes, discoloration, or abnormal growth patterns. Correctly identify pests to determine the best management techniques. Use field guides, internet resources, or local extension offices to identify common garden pests and distinguish between beneficial and hazardous insects.

2. Cultural Controls: Use cultural methods to help reduce pest and disease issues in the garden. Crop rotation, companion planting, correct spacing, and soil management

are all practices that serve to disrupt insect life cycles, reduce pest populations, and enhance plant health. Choose disease-resistant plant varieties wherever feasible to decrease your vulnerability to common garden ailments.

3. Biological Controls: Use natural predators, parasites, or diseases to regulate pest populations in your garden. Encourage beneficial insects like ladybugs, lacewings, predatory beetles, and parasitic wasps by providing habitat, shelter, and nectar. Introduce helpful nematodes, predatory mites, or microbial pesticides to target specific pest species while protecting beneficial organisms.

4. Mechanical Controls: To manage garden pests and illnesses, use physical or mechanical methods. To minimize pest numbers, handpick caterpillars, aphids, and snails and properly dispose of them. Install barriers such as row covers, netting, or screens to keep pests away from vulnerable plants or prevent them from accessing fruits and vegetables. Use traps, sticky traps, or pheromone traps to keep track of pest populations and catch them before they cause damage, use traps, sticky traps, or pheromone traps.

5. Chemical Controls: Only use chemical pesticides as a last option to manage serious pest or disease outbreaks. Choose low-toxicity insecticides that target specific pests while causing little harm to beneficial creatures, animals, and the environment. When spraying pesticides, carefully follow the label directions and use suitable protective equipment to reduce exposure and danger to human health.

6. Monitoring and Prevention: Check plants on a regular basis for symptoms of insect infestation or disease, and respond quickly to any issues that occur. Inspect plants for pests, illnesses, or stress symptoms, and treat them early to prevent the problem from spreading. To eliminate pest and disease reservoirs, maintain proper garden cleanliness by removing plant detritus, falling leaves, and unhealthy plant material.

7. Integrated Pest Management (IPM): Use an integrated pest management (IPM) approach that integrates many tactics to efficiently manage pests and illnesses. Incorporate cultural, biological, mechanical, and chemical controls into a complete pest management program. Monitor pest populations, monitor plant health, and alter treatment

strategies to meet your garden's individual needs and conditions.

8. Education and Awareness: Attend workshops, seminars, or instructional programs to learn more about common garden pests, illnesses, and management approaches. Consult with local gardening experts, master gardeners, or extension agents for specialized ideas and help. Share your expertise and resources with other gardeners in order to develop community-wide, sustainable pest and disease management strategies.

Gardeners who use proactive pest and disease control practices may limit the impact of pests and diseases on their plants, reduce their dependency on chemical pesticides, and build a healthy and resilient garden environment. Implementing integrated pest management (IPM) concepts maintains ecological balance, conserves natural resources, and encourages long-term success and pleasure in the garden.

CHAPTER 8

Harvesting and Enjoying Your Garden

Harvesting and enjoying the rewards of your effort is one of the most satisfying elements of gardening. Whether you're harvesting fresh veggies, herbs, fruits, or flowers, taking the time to appreciate your garden's bounty and beauty provides you with delight and satisfaction.

Here's a full guide to harvesting and enjoying your garden:
1. Harvest fruits, vegetables, herbs, and flowers when they are fully ripe for the optimum flavor, texture, and nutritional value. Monitor plants on a regular basis and harvest when fruits are totally mature, veggies are delicate, herbs are fragrant, and flowers are in full bloom. Check the harvesting rules for each plant species to guarantee the best time and quality.

2. Harvesting Techniques: Use sharp, clean gardening tools like scissors, pruners, or a harvesting knife to harvest crops effectively and with minimal plant damage. Cut fruits, vegetables, and herbs off the plant using a clean, straight cut

to avoid ripping or bruising. Handle fragile flowers gently to prevent harming the petals or stems.

3. Harvesting Methods: Harvest crops individually by handpicking or cutting them from the plant, or harvest entire plants for higher yields or to make way for succession planting. Collect picked food in baskets, buckets, or trays and preserve it fresh until ready to use or store. To enhance freshness and flavor, harvest in the early morning or evening when temperatures are lower.

4. Post-Harvest Handling: To minimize bruising or damage during transportation or storage, handle harvested food carefully. Harvested crops should be free of debris, soil, and plant material and lightly rinsed with water to eliminate dirt and residue. Sort and examine the collected produce for quality, rejecting any damaged, diseased, or overripe products.

5. Storage and Preservation: Properly store gathered food to ensure freshness and shelf life. Refrigerate perishable crops like leafy greens, herbs, and berries in plastic bags or containers with air holes to keep them wet and avoid wilting. To extend the storage life of root crops, such as onions and

garlic, keep them in a cold, dry, and dark environment, such as a root cellar or pantry. Canning, freezing, drying, or pickling fruits and vegetables allows you to store them for a long time and enjoy them later.

6. Culinary Creations: Get creative with your garden harvests by mixing fresh, local veggies into delectable dishes and dinners. Experiment with various flavors, textures, and combinations to highlight the variety and richness of your garden vegetables. Enjoy garden-fresh salads, soups, stir-fries, sauces, and desserts cooked with ripe, aromatic items from the garden.

7. Sharing and Community: Share your garden's harvest with friends, family, neighbors, and community members to share joy and create relationships. Host garden parties, potluck dinners, or food swaps to share your produce and culinary talents. Donate any extra crops to local food banks, shelters, or community organizations to help those in need and create food security in your area.

8. Garden Enjoyment: Whether you're harvesting, tending plants, or simply lounging outside, take the time to appreciate the beauty and peace of your garden. Admire the

bright blossoms, inhale pleasant smells, listen to birdsong, and feel the ground beneath your feet. Embrace gardening's therapeutic advantages, as well as the sense of success and contentment that comes from maintaining and growing your own natural space.

Knowing When to Harvest

Knowing when to harvest is critical for increasing the flavor, nutritional value, and overall quality of your garden food. Harvesting at the appropriate time ensures that fruits, vegetables, herbs, and flowers are at their full maturity and ready for consumption.

Here's a full explanation of when to harvest different sorts of crops:

1. Vegetables: Root Vegetables: Harvest carrots, beets, radishes, and potatoes when they are the right size and color. Gently remove the dirt at the plant's base and lift its roots to check their size and health. Leafy Greens: Harvest lettuce, spinach, kale, and Swiss chard while they are fresh, tender, and bright green. Harvest the outer leaves as required, or trim the entire plant back to promote new growth.

Tomatoes: Harvest tomatoes when they are full color and firm, depending on the type. Ripe tomatoes should have a consistent color, a firm firmness, and a small give when gently pressed. Avoid harvesting tomatoes that are too green or firm.

Peppers: Harvest when they are mature in size, color, and flavor. Most peppers mature from green to red, yellow, orange, or purple. Pick peppers that are firm, shiny, and completely colored.

Beans: Pick the beans when they are fresh, fragile, and snap readily when bent. Pick beans on a regular basis to ensure consistent production and avoid overripe pods.

Cucumbers: Harvest them when they are firm, crisp, and consistently green. Pick cucumbers before they ripen or turn yellow.

2. Fruits: Berries: Pick strawberries, raspberries, blueberries, and blackberries when they are completely ripe and readily detached from the plant with a little tug. Ripe berries should be plump, juicy, and colorful. Melons: Harvest watermelons, cantaloupes, and honeydews when they have a

delicious scent, change color, and exhibit symptoms of maturity (dull skin, yellowing on the underside).

Apples: Harvest apples when they are completely ripe and easily remove them from the tree with a little twist. Ripe apples should have a bright color, a firm texture, and a pleasant flavor.

Stone Fruits: Harvest peaches, plums, cherries, and apricots when they reach their peak color, size, and flavor. Ripe stone fruits should be somewhat soft to the touch and easy to remove from the tree or limb.

3. Herbs: Leafy Herbs: Harvest basil, cilantro, parsley, and mint when they are lush, fragrant, and flavorful. Pinch or clip individual leaves or stems as needed, or prune entire plants to encourage bushy growth. Woody

Herbs: Harvest woody herbs like rosemary, thyme, sage, and oregano while they are actively growing and have plenty of leaves. Trim stems and branches as needed, but avoid excessive pruning, which can damage the plant.

3. Flowers: Cut Flowers: Pick cut flowers like roses, dahlias, zinnias, and sunflowers when they are

completely open, vivid, and free of pests and illnesses. Cut stems at an angle with sharp scissors or pruners and immerse them immediately in water to keep them fresh.

4. General Tips: Check for maturity: Use visual cues, texture, smell, and taste to assess the maturity of fruits, vegetables, herbs, and flowers. Each crop has its own set of maturity signs, so get to know each plant's unique qualities.

5. Harvest Frequently: Harvest crops on a frequent basis to avoid over-ripening, bolting, and spoiling. Check plants regularly during peak harvest periods and collect food as soon as they reach the appropriate level of maturity. Handle Harvested Produce gently to avoid bruising, damage, and premature spoilage. To ensure maximum quality and longevity, use clean, sharp equipment and treat fragile crops with caution. Knowing when to harvest and paying attention to each crop's distinct features will allow you to enjoy the freshest, most tasty, and most healthy vegetables from your garden. Harvesting at the correct time helps you enjoy the

bounty of your garden and make the most of your efforts.

Harvesting Techniques

Harvesting processes vary according to the crop and its qualities.

Here's a comprehensive summary of harvesting strategies for several sorts of crops:

1. Hand harvesting: Many fruits, vegetables, herbs, and flowers are hand-gathered, either individually or in small groups. To avoid plant damage, make clean cuts with sharp, clean gardening scissors, pruners, or shears. With one hand, hold the plant's stem or branch while using the other to snip or pinch off individual fruits, veggies, or flowers. Handle delicate crops like berries or herbs gently to prevent bruising or crushing.

2. Cutting: Some crops must be chopped rather than pulled or twisted to prevent damage to the plant or surrounding foliage. Cut cleanly at the stem or branch base with a sharp knife, pruning shears, or scissors. Cut stems at an angle to

improve water absorption and extend the freshness of harvested vegetables.

3. Twisting: To harvest some crops, such as tomatoes, peppers, and eggplants, twist or gently tug the fruit until it separates from the plant. Hold the fruit in one hand and twist or spin it with the other until it is free of the stem. Avoid pulling too forcefully or with excessive effort, since this might harm the plant or cause the fruit to bruise.

4. Snapping: To harvest snap beans, peas, and other legumes, gently bend the pod until it breaks at its natural breaking point. With one hand, hold the stem or branch while using the other to break off individual pods, ensuring they are young, sensitive, and crisp.

5. Pulling: Root vegetables, including carrots, radishes, and beets, are hand-harvested. Using one hand, firmly grab the leaf or top of the root, and with the other, carefully pull the vegetable out of the earth. Avoid tugging or yanking too hard on the plant, since this might harm the roots or snap off the leaves.

6. Shaking: To remove mature fruits or seeds from a plant, shake or lightly tap it. Gently shake or tap the plant, holding

a container or tarp below to catch any falling fruits or seeds. Avoid shaking too forcefully, since this might harm the plant or cause immature fruits or seeds to fall prematurely.

7. Brushing: Harvest certain crops, such as raspberries or blackberries, by gently brushing or combing the fruits off the plant with your fingertips or a specialized instrument. With one hand, hold the stem or branch while using the other to brush or comb through the fruit clusters, enabling ripe fruits to fall into the container below.

8. Timing: Harvest vegetables at the peak of maturity for the optimum flavor, texture, and nutritional value. Check plants on a regular basis and harvest crops as soon as they reach maturity to avoid over-ripeness, bolting, and spoilage. By may improve the quality, freshness, and lifespan of your garden food by harvesting it correctly and handling it with care. Take the time to harvest vegetables at their peak maturity and reap the many benefits of your gardening efforts.

Storing Your Harvest

Preserving your crop allows you to enjoy the bounty of your garden all year by prolonging the shelf life of fresh food and making tasty homemade preserves.

Here's a full description of the many ways to preserve your harvest:

1. **Canning:** Canning is a common way to preserve fruits, vegetables, jams, jellies, sauces, and pickles in sealed jars or cans. To properly process low- or high-acid foods, use a water bath canner or a pressure canner. For safe and successful preservation, use established recipes and canning recommendations from recognized sources. Before filling jars with prepared food, sterilize the jars, lids, and bands, and then process them in boiling water or a pressure canner for the specified periods and pressures. For long-term storage, keep canned products in a cold, dark, and dry location, and inspect jars on a regular basis for indications of rotting.

2. **Freezing:** Freezing is a simple and effective way to preserve fruits, vegetables, herbs, and prepared goods. Blanch veggies briefly in boiling water, then immediately

chill in ice water before draining and packing for freezing. Place fruits, vegetables, and herbs in freezer-safe containers or bags, eliminating extra air to avoid freezer burn. Label containers with the contents and the date of freezing, and keep them in the freezer at 0°F (-18°C) or below for best results. Use frozen produce within the prescribed storage durations for the greatest flavor and texture, and avoid refreezing thawed products.

3. **Drying:** Drying, or dehydration, is a traditional way of preserving fruits, vegetables, herbs, and meats by eliminating moisture from them. Dry foods at low temperatures using a dehydrator, oven, or air-drying technique until crisp and leathery. Place sliced or chopped vegetables in a single layer on drying trays, spreading them evenly to facilitate air circulation. To keep dried foods away from moisture and pests, store them in airtight containers or bags in a cold, dark, and dry area. Rehydrate dried items as needed by soaking them in water or broth before cooking or eating.

4. **Fermenting:** Fermentation is a natural preservation mechanism in which beneficial bacteria or yeast convert

carbohydrates into acids, alcohols, or gases. Use fermentation to create sauerkraut, kimchi, pickles, yogurt, kefir, kombucha, and sourdough bread. Season vegetables, fruits, or dairy products with salt, brine, or starter cultures, and then let them ferment at room temperature for a few days to weeks. Regularly monitor fermentation progress and taste samples to assess flavor development and readiness. To delay fermentation and keep fermented foods fresh, store them in the refrigerator or in a cold, dark spot.

5. **Pickling:** Pickling is a food preservation technique that involves immersing items in a brine or acidic solution to preserve them and produce sour, tasty pickles. To produce pickling brine, combine vinegar, salt, sugar, and spices, and then pour it over prepared vegetables, fruits, or eggs in sterilized jars. To properly seal jars, process them in a water bath canner using the specified periods and temperatures. Let pickles cure for several weeks to develop flavor before eating, and keep them in a cold, dark area for long-term preservation.

6. **Root cellaring:** Root cellaring is a traditional way of preserving root vegetables, squash, onions, garlic, and other

hardy crops in a cool, damp environment. Store harvested crops in a root cellar, basement, garage, or insulated storage room with temperatures ranging from 32°F to 40°F (0°C to 4°C) and high humidity. Store crops in bins, crates, or mesh bags to promote air circulation and avoid rotting or sprouting. Regularly inspect stored produce for symptoms of rotting or decay, and discard any damaged or rotten goods to avoid spread.

7. **Preserving herbs:** To preserve fresh herbs, dry them, freeze them, infuse them with oil or vinegar, or make herb-infused salts or sugars. To dry herbs, hang them in bundles or spread them on screens in a warm, well-ventilated room until crisp and dry. Finely chop herbs and place them in ice cube trays with water or oil to freeze. Once frozen, transfer the cubes to freezer bags for storage. Season salads, marinades, sauces, and dressings with herb-infused oils or vinegars, or sprinkle herb-infused salts or sugars over cooked meals for extra flavor.

8. **Jam and Jelly Making:** Preserve fruits and berries by preparing homemade jams, jellies, preserves, or fruit spreads. Cook the fruit with sugar, pectin, and acid until it

thickens to a spreadable consistency, then transfer it to sterilized jars and seal with lids. For short-term storage, process jars in a boiling water bath or chill them before storing them in the refrigerator. Try homemade jams and jellies over toast, biscuits, pancakes, yogurt, or as fillings for pastries and desserts. By combining these preservation methods, you can maximize your garden production and enjoy fresh, tasty vegetables all year. Experiment with various techniques and recipes.

CHAPTER 9

Cooking with Garden-Fresh Produce

Cooking with garden-fresh food allows you to incorporate the tastes and nutritional advantages of homegrown fruits, vegetables, herbs, and spices into tasty and healthy meals. Whether you're collecting ripe tomatoes, crisp lettuce, aromatic herbs, or vibrant peppers, there are many ways to integrate garden food into your recipes.

Here's a full guide to cooking using garden-fresh produce:

1. **Fresh salads:** Create vivid salads using garden-fresh lettuce, spinach, arugula, or mixed greens as the foundation, then top with colorful veggies, fruits, nuts, seeds, and protein-rich toppings. For crunch and flavor, throw in diced tomatoes, cucumbers, carrots, bell peppers, radishes, or avocados. Serve with homemade vinaigrettes or creamy dressings prepared with fresh herbs and citrus. For a refreshing snack or side dish, garnish salads with herbs like basil, parsley, cilantro, dill, or mint.

2. **Garden-fresh salsas and dips:** Make delectable salsas and dips using fresh tomatoes, onions, peppers, cilantro, and jalapenos from your garden. To prepare classic salsa fresca or Pico de Gallo, mix chopped tomatoes, onions, peppers, cilantro, and lime juice. Serve with tortilla chips, tacos, quesadillas, or grilled meats. To prepare creamy guacamole, combine ripe avocados, garlic, lime juice, cilantro, and jalapenos. Serve as a dip or topping for tacos, nachos, or sandwiches.

3. **Grilled vegetables:** Grill garden-fresh veggies like zucchini, eggplant, bell peppers, onions, mushrooms, and asparagus to bring out their natural flavors and caramelize. Brush veggies with olive oil, season with salt, pepper, and herbs like rosemary, thyme, or oregano, then grill over medium heat until soft and gently browned. For a blast of smoky flavor and texture, serve grilled veggies as a side dish, mix with pasta or salads, or stack over sandwiches, pizzas, or wraps.

4. **Herbaceous Pastas with Pesto:** Make herbaceous pasta recipes using garden-fresh herbs like basil, parsley, cilantro, and mint. Toss cooked pasta with homemade pesto made

from fresh basil, garlic, pine nuts, Parmesan cheese, and olive oil; serve with cherry tomatoes, roasted veggies, or grilled chicken. To enhance flavor and scent, garnish pasta dishes with chopped herbs and grated cheese. Serve as a delightful main course or side dish.

5. **Garden Fresh Soups and Stews:** Make hearty soups and stews using garden-fresh veggies, herbs, and legumes for a satisfying and healthy supper. Simmer chopped tomatoes, onions, carrots, celery, potatoes, and beans in vegetable or chicken broth with fresh herbs like thyme, bay leaves, or parsley until the veggies are soft and the flavors blend. Serve garden-fresh soups and stews with crusty bread, crackers, or a side salad for a nutritious and fulfilling dinner that highlights the season's tastes.

6. **Fresh Herbal Garnishes and Infusions:** Use fresh herbs from the garden as garnishes and infusions to improve the flavor and presentation of your dishes. For a burst of color and flavor, sprinkle chopped herbs like basil, cilantro, dill, or chives over completed meals. Serve with a slice of lemon or lime for extra freshness. Infuse oils, vinegars, or spirits with fresh herbs and spices to make flavorful condiments,

marinades, or cocktail mixers that will enhance the flavor of your dishes.

7. **Garden Fresh Desserts:** Use garden-fresh fruits like berries, peaches, apples, and figs to make wonderful sweets like pies, tarts, and crisps, cobblers, or fruit salads. Make seasonal fruit pies or tarts using handmade pie crust and fresh fruit filling, then serve with whipped cream or vanilla ice cream. Make fruit salads with a mix of garden-fresh fruits, mint, and a drizzle of honey or citrus juice for a light and delicious dessert. Cooking with garden-fresh food allows you to enjoy the flavors, textures, and fragrances of seasonal crops while also creating tasty and healthy meals that highlight the garden's bounty. Experiment with different recipes, tastes, and cooking methods to get the most out of your homegrown produce and savor the taste of freshly gathered deliciousness in every bite.

CHAPTER 10

Troubleshooting Common Garden Issues

Troubleshooting common garden issues is an important skill for keeping plants healthy and fruitful. By detecting and treating problems as soon as possible, you may avoid harm, stimulate plant development, and optimize garden output. Here's a full summary of typical garden issues and solutions:

1. Pests: Identify common garden pests like aphids, caterpillars, beetles, and mites by monitoring plants on a regular basis for evidence of damage, pests, or eggs. Use integrated pest management (IPM) strategies to efficiently manage pest populations, including cultural, biological, mechanical, and least-toxic insecticides. Encourage natural predators such as ladybugs, lacewings, birds, and beneficial insects to help manage pest numbers organically. Keep an eye out for insect activity on your plants and respond early to keep infestations from spreading and causing serious harm.

2. Diseases: Identify common garden diseases such as powdery mildew, blight, rust, and damping-off by looking for signs like wilting, yellowing, spotting, or mold development on leaves, stems, or fruits. Maintain proper garden hygiene by removing sick plant material, fallen leaves, and debris to lessen disease pressure and avoid pathogen transmission. Provide enough air circulation, spacing, and drainage to minimize humidity and produce an unfavorable environment for fungal and bacterial illnesses. Plant disease-resistant plant kinds wherever feasible, and avoid growing sensitive crops in the same spot year after year.

3. Nutrient deficiencies: Identify nutritional shortages like nitrogen, phosphorus, potassium, calcium, magnesium, or iron by looking for signs like yellowing leaves, stunted growth, poor fruit set, or leaf discoloration. Perform a soil test to determine nutrient levels and pH balance, then amend the soil as necessary to rectify deficiencies or imbalances. Use balanced fertilization with organic or synthetic fertilizers to restore nutrients and encourage healthy plant development. Add organic matter to the soil to promote fertility, structure, and nutrient availability.

4. Environmental stress: Identify environmental stresses such as severe temperatures, drought, waterlogging, poor soil drainage, or insufficient sunshine by looking for plant signs like wilting, leaf burn, or leaf drop. Provide adequate irrigation, mulching, and shade to reduce temperature extremes and provide ideal growth conditions for plants. Add organic matter like compost, perlite, or vermiculite to heavy clay or compacted soil to improve its structure and drainage. To reduce stress and enhance plant resilience, choose plant kinds that are well-suited to your local climate, soil conditions, and sunshine exposure.

5. Weeds: Identify typical garden weeds such as dandelions, crabgrass, chickweed, and purslane based on their growth tendencies, leaf forms, and reproductive systems. Use preventive measures like mulching, weed barriers, or cover crops to reduce weed development and prevent weed seeds from germinating. To avoid competing with garden plants for water, nutrients, and sunshine, remove weeds as soon as possible by hand-pulling, hoeing, or cultivating shallowly. To reduce soil disturbance and prevent weed seed dissemination, mulch or cover exposed soil with a thick planting of desired plants.

6. Animal Damage: Identify common garden pests, including deer, rabbits, squirrels, birds, and rodents, by looking for indications of feeding damage, footprints, or droppings in the garden. Use physical barriers like fences, netting, or row covers to keep animals out of the garden and sensitive plants safe from browsing or predation. Use repellents or deterrents, such as scent deterrents, visual scare devices, or motion-activated sprinklers, to keep animals out of your garden.

Harvest crops immediately and remove any fallen fruits or vegetables to eliminate food sources and animal attraction. You can keep your garden healthy and growing by systematically analyzing common problems and adopting effective remedies. To watchful, study plant behavior, and handle difficulties as soon as possible to avoid problems worsening and ensure the success of your gardening activities.

Identifying Plant Diseases

Identifying plant diseases is critical for your garden's health and production. Recognizing typical symptoms and indicators of illness allows you to take proper action to avoid pathogen spread and reduce plant damage.

Here's a full explanation of how to diagnose plant diseases:

1. Visual symptoms: Leaf Symptoms: Check for discoloration, wilting, yellowing, browning, or spotting on leaves. Depending on the illness, symptoms might take the form of lesions, necrosis, chlorosis, or mottling.

Stem Symptoms: Look for lesions, cankers, edema, gallstones, or discoloration on stems. Check for symptoms of wilting, dieback, or stem collapse, which might suggest vascular disease or fungal infection.

Root Symptoms: Check the roots for rotting, decay, discoloration, or necrosis. Nematodes or soil-borne diseases can cause stunted growth, root galls, or root knots. Look for these signs.

Fruit Symptoms: Examine fruits for mold, rot, lesions, flaws, and abnormalities. Look for symptoms of fungal, bacterial, or viral illnesses that cause early ripening, fruit loss, or reduced production.

Flower Symptoms: Inspect flowers for wilting, discoloration, distortion, or irregular growth. Pathogens or environmental stresses can cause floral blight, petal spots, or blossom abortion. Look for these indicators.

2. Signs of infection: Fungal Growth: Check for powdery mildew, downy mildew, mold, or fungal spores on the leaves, stems, or fruits. Fungal growth might manifest as white, gray, black, or colorful patches, granules, or threads.

Bacterial Oozing: Look for bacterial ooze, slime, or exudate on stems, leaves, and fruit surfaces. Bacterial infections can create slimy or watery sores, cankers, and sticky or foul-smelling oozing.

Pest Infestation: Check plants for evidence of pest damage, such as chewing, mining, sucking, or piercing of leaves, stems, or fruits. Look for pest eggs, larvae, nymphs, and adults on plant surfaces or in the soil.

3. Environmental conditions: Take into account environmental parameters, including temperature, humidity, moisture, light, soil conditions, and air movement, which can all contribute to disease development. Keep an eye on weather patterns, watering methods, and seasonal changes that might produce an environment conducive to pathogen growth. Identify disease-predisposition patterns, such as certain plant species, planting areas, or cultural practices.

4. Disease Diagnosis: Use gardening materials, extension publications, or internet databases to identify common plant diseases based on symptoms, signs, and plant type. Take images or samples of afflicted plants, such as leaves, stems, roots, fruits, or flowers, to ensure an accurate diagnosis by local extension agents, plant pathologists, or gardening specialists. Using diagnostic equipment such as hand lenses, microscopes, or diagnostic kits, examine plant tissues, pathogens, or disease vectors to confirm disease presence.

5. Prevention and Management: Maintain proper garden hygiene by removing sick plant material, fallen leaves, and debris to limit disease reservoirs and prevent pathogen transmission. Use cultural techniques, including crop rotation, correct spacing, and soil management, to boost plant health and reduce disease pressure. To limit susceptibility to common plant diseases, use resistant plant types, disease-free seeds, or certified nursery stock. Use fungicides, bactericides, or biological treatments to protect plants and manage disease outbreaks.

You can keep your garden healthy and robust by recognizing plant diseases early on and adopting proactive efforts to avoid and treat them. Stay watchful, examine plants on a regular basis, and apply suitable solutions to reduce disease effects on your garden plants while increasing growth and output.

Pest management

Pest management Gardeners face continuous difficulty in dealing with pests, but there are numerous successful ways for regulating insect populations and preserving their plants. Using integrated pest management (IPM) approaches, you can reduce your use of chemical pesticides while also promoting a healthy and balanced environment in your garden.

Here's a complete guide to dealing with pests in your garden:

1. **Identify pests:** Check plants on a regular basis for symptoms of pest damage, such as chewed leaves, stippled foliage, curled or deformed growth, fruit holes, or insect activity on the plant. Identify common garden pests such as aphids, caterpillars, beetles, mites, slugs, snails, and rodents based on their size, shape, color, behavior, and eating patterns. Use gardening materials, field guides, or internet databases to identify pests based on their appearance, life cycle, and host plants.

2. **Monitor pest populations:** Use sticky traps, pheromone traps, or visual inspections to monitor insect numbers and determine the severity of infestations. Inspect plants on a regular basis for eggs, larvae, nymphs, or adult insects, and keep track of your findings to monitor pest activity over time. Keep an eye on environmental factors, including temperature, humidity, rainfall, and seasonal changes, since they can all have an impact on insect numbers and plant vulnerability.

3. **Implement cultural controls.** Maintain proper garden cleanliness by eliminating weeds, trash, fallen leaves, and plant remnants that might attract pests or serve as breeding grounds. Use crop rotation, companion planting, and intercropping to disrupt pest lifecycles, attract beneficial insects, and keep pests away from vulnerable plants. Maintain ideal plant growth conditions by ensuring adequate soil fertility, hydration, pH balance, and sunshine exposure to improve plant health and insect resistance.

4. **Use biological controls:** Use natural enemies like predatory insects, parasitic wasps, and beneficial nematodes to manage pest populations and preserve ecological balance

in your garden. to attract beneficial insects, grow nectar-rich flowers, create insect hotels, or provide habitat such as hedgerows, cover crops, and mulch. Use biological control agents like ladybugs, lacewings, predatory mites, and parasitic wasps to target and reduce pest populations.

5. **Use mechanical controls:** Remove pests from plants by hand-picking, trapping, or vacuuming them, especially bigger pests like caterpillars, beetles, and slugs. Use physical barriers, such as row coverings, netting, or screens, to keep pests away from susceptible plants and host crops. Use physical obstacles such as fences, barriers, or traps to keep bigger pests like deer, rabbits, and rats out of your garden and inflicting damage.

6. **Use the least toxic pesticides:** To reduce pest infestations, use the least hazardous pesticides possible, such as insecticidal soaps, neem oil, horticultural oils, or herbal insecticides. Use insecticides sparingly, following label directions for timing and dose, to efficiently target pests while minimizing non-target effects. Rotate pesticide classes, active chemicals, or modes of action to avoid insect resistance and ensure efficacy over time.

7. **Practice Integrated Pest Management (IPM):** Implement a comprehensive IPM program that includes several pest management tactics, including cultural, biological, mechanical, and chemical treatments, to reduce pest damage and protect plant health. Regularly monitor pest populations, determine intervention thresholds, and choose the most effective management measures based on pest biology, environmental circumstances, and plant vulnerability. Document pest management operations, monitor results, and adapt techniques as needed to ensure long-term pest control and reduce dependency on chemical pesticides. By taking a proactive and comprehensive approach to pest control, you can effectively manage pest populations, protect your plants from harm, and foster a healthy and productive garden environment. Stay educated, examine plants on a regular basis, respond quickly to pest outbreaks, and keep your garden ecology balanced.

CHAPTER 11

Soil and Nutrient Issues

Soil and nutrient concerns can have an impact on plant growth, health, and production in the garden. Understanding typical soil issues and nutrient deficits allows you to take actions to increase soil fertility, structure, and nutrient availability, resulting in healthier plant development.

Here's a full review of soil and nutrient problems and how to solve them:

1. **Soil pH imbalance:** Use a soil test kit or send a soil sample to a competent laboratory to evaluate whether the pH is too acidic (below 6.0) or too alkaline (above 7.5). Depending on plant requirements and soil test recommendations, amend acidic soil using lime to increase pH or acidic fertilizers such as sulfur to decrease pH. Gradually adjust soil pH over time to minimize shock to plants or disruption of soil microbial activity.

2. **Poor soil drainage:** promote soil drainage by adding organic matter like compost, aged manure, or shredded

leaves to heavy clay or compacted soil to promote structure and water penetration. Use raised beds, berms, or French drains to divert excess water away from flooded regions and create well-drained planting beds for garden plants. Avoid overwatering plants and let the soil dry between waterings to avoid soggy conditions that encourage root rot, fungal infections, and nutrient leaching.

3. **Nutrient deficiencies:** Perform a soil test to determine nutrient levels and discover deficits in critical elements including nitrogen (N), phosphorus (P), potassium (K), calcium (Ca), magnesium (Mg), sulfur (S), iron (Fe), zinc (Zn), manganese (Mn), and boron (B). Based on soil test results, add organic fertilizers, compost, or mineral additions to restore depleted nutrients and boost soil fertility. Use balanced fertilizers with the proper NPK ratios or specialty fertilizers to treat particular nutrient deficits and promote healthy plant growth and development.

4. **Nutrient imbalances:** Maintain optimum nutrient balance in the soil by using fertilizers in suitable amounts and avoiding overuse of single nutrients, which can disrupt nutrient absorption or produce toxicity. Use slow-release

fertilizers, organic amendments, or nutrient-rich compost to offer a consistent supply of nutrients to plants throughout time, lowering the danger of nutritional imbalances. Monitor plant development, leaf color, and general health for signs of nutrient imbalances such as chlorosis, stunted growth, leaf tip burn, or leaf curling, and adjust fertilizer as needed.

5. **Soil compaction:** To enhance soil structure and porosity, aerate compacted soil with mechanical aerators, hand tools, or organic materials like compost, gypsum, or perlite. Avoid using high-foot traffic or machinery on garden beds, walks, or planting areas to minimize soil compaction and maintain soil tilt and friability. Add cover crops, green manures, or mulch to the soil to boost organic matter content, improve soil aggregation, and improve tilth and drainage over time.

6. **Soil Erosion:** To stabilize soil and minimize topsoil loss, employ erosion management methods such as contour planting, terracing, mulching, and erosion barriers. Plant erosion-resistant ground coverings, shrubs, or trees on slopes or exposed places to anchor soil, minimize runoff, and prevent wind and water erosion. Keep vegetative cover, plant permanent vegetation, or use erosion control blankets

or mats to protect bare soil surfaces and enhance soil stability and conservation.

7. **Soil salinity:** Measure soil salinity using an electrical conductivity (EC) meter or send a soil sample to a competent laboratory to determine soluble salts and soil salinity levels. Use water to flush salt-affected soils, allowing excess salts to sink below the root zone and gradually improving soil drainage and salinity. Avoid over-fertilization with high-salt fertilizers or excessive use of saline irrigation water, which can increase soil salinity and negatively impact plant development and health. By proactively addressing soil and nutrient concerns and using proper soil management strategies, you may enhance soil fertility, structure, and health while also providing ideal growth conditions for garden plants. Regular soil testing, monitoring, and management are essential for diagnosing and addressing soil and nutrient issues, as well as maintaining your garden's long-term production and sustainability.

Environmental Factors

Environmental elements are important in gardening since they may have a substantial influence on plant growth, health, and output. Understanding how environmental factors such as temperature, sunshine, water, humidity, wind, and climate affect plants will help you produce ideal growing conditions and increase garden success.

Here's a comprehensive overview of environmental elements in gardening:

1. Temperature: Different plants require different temperatures to germinate, develop, blossom, and fruit. Keep an eye on temperature swings and extremes, such as frost, heatwaves, and temperature changes, since they can stress plants and impair development. Select plant species that are appropriate for your climate, and consider utilizing season extenders such as row covers, cloches, or cold frames to protect plants from temperature extremes.

2. Sunlight: Sunlight is required for photosynthesis, the process by which plants transform light energy into chemical energy that fuels growth and development. Assess your

garden's solar exposure and choose plants that demand full sun, medium shade, or complete shade. Allow enough sun exposure for sun-loving plants like tomatoes, peppers, and herbs, while providing shade or filtered light for shade-tolerant plants like lettuce, spinach, and Cole crops.

3. Water: Water is essential for plant development, nutrient absorption, and cellular activity; yet, inadequate or excessive water can stress plants, causing wilting, dehydration, or root rot. Monitor soil moisture levels on a regular basis and water plants deeply and rarely to promote deep root development and drought resistance. Use mulch, drip irrigation, or soaker hoses to keep soil wet, control weeds, and limit water evaporation from the soil surface.

4. Humidity: Humidity levels impact transpiration, or the process by which plants lose moisture via their leaves, as well as plant water intake and development. Keep an eye on humidity levels both indoors and outdoors, especially in greenhouses or humid locations where high humidity can lead to fungal illnesses and insect infestations. Use fans, vents, or dehumidifiers to maintain ideal humidity levels and minimize plant stress.

5. Wind: Wind may dehydrate plants, inflict mechanical damage, and impede pollination, especially in exposed or windy areas. To protect plants from severe winds, use windbreaks such as fences, hedges, or windbreak barriers. These will produce microclimates that provide protection and minimize wind stress. Stake tall or top-heavy plants, fasten trellises, and build support systems to avoid wind damage and keep plants stable in windy weather.

6. Climate: Climate refers to long-term weather patterns, such as temperature, precipitation, humidity, wind, and sunshine, that affect plant development and adaptability. When planning and planting your garden, choose plant kinds that are suited to your local environment, taking into account hardiness zones, frost dates, and growth seasons. Adjust gardening methods, crop choices, and planting dates to account for seasonal changes and weather variables such as drought, heatwaves, or cold snaps.

7. Pollution and contaminants: Pollutants in the environment, including air and water pollution, soil contamination, and chemical residues, can have an impact on plant and food safety. Reduce your exposure to

contaminants by practicing organic gardening, avoiding polluted soils or water sources, and employing natural or low-impact pest management techniques. Test soil, water, and plant tissues for pollutants, heavy metals, and harmful compounds, and take corrective measures to protect plant and human health.

Seasonal Gardening Tips

Seasonal gardening advice may help you get the most out of each season, optimize plant development, and increase garden production all year. By may create a flourishing garden and get an abundant harvest by modifying gardening methods, planting schedules, and maintenance duties in response to seasonal variations.

Here's a comprehensive list of seasonal gardening suggestions for each season:

Spring Gardening Tips:

1. Prepare Garden Beds: Remove waste, weeds, and detritus from garden beds, then treat soil with compost, organic matter, and balanced fertilizer to replace nutrients and enhance soil structure.

2. Start Seeds Indoors: For warm-season crops like tomatoes, peppers, eggplants, and cucumbers, start seeds indoors using seed trays, grow lights, and heat mats to encourage germination and seedling growth.

3. Harden off Seedlings: Allow seedlings to adjust to outside circumstances over several days by exposing them to

sunshine, wind, and temperature variations before transplanting them into the garden.

4. Plant Cool-Season Crops: As soon as soil temperatures allow, sow seeds or transplant seedlings of cool-season crops like lettuce, spinach, kale, carrots, peas, and radishes into the garden.

5. Monitor weather forecasts and use row covers, cloches, or frost blankets to protect fragile plants from late frosts or cold snaps, which can harm developing foliage and blooms.

Summer gardening tips:

1. Water Plants deeply and consistently: To maintain soil moisture levels during hot and dry weather, focus on the root zone and minimize overhead watering to reduce evaporation and foliar disease.

2. Mulch Beds: To conserve moisture, suppress weeds, and regulate soil temperature during the hot summer months, cover garden beds with organic mulch such as straw, shredded leaves, or grass clippings.

3. Install shade cloth, umbrellas, or temporary structures to protect heat-sensitive plants, seedlings, and container gardens from direct sunlight and high temperatures.

4. Harvest frequently: On a regular basis, harvest fruits, vegetables, herbs, and flowers to ensure ongoing production, minimize over-ripening or bolting, and promote the development of new growth and blossoms.

5. Monitor Pests and Diseases: Inspect plants on a regular basis for signs of pest infestations, fungal diseases, or nutrient deficiencies, and take immediate action to control pests, apply fungicides, or adjust fertilization as needed.

Fall Gardening Tips:

1. Sow seeds or transplant seedlings of cool-season crops like broccoli, cauliflower, cabbage, Brussels sprouts, and kale into your garden for fall and winter harvests.

2. Extend the growing season by installing cold frames, hoop houses, or row covers, which will protect tender plants from early frosts and allow for continued harvests well into the fall.

3. Harvest and Preserve: Gather mature fruits, vegetables, and herbs before frost and can, freeze, dry, or ferment excess harvests to enjoy garden-fresh produce all winter.

4. Clean up garden beds by removing spent crops, weeds, and debris, then adding a layer of compost, mulch, or cover crops to replenish soil nutrients, suppress weeds, and protect soil from erosion over the winter.

5. Plant Bulbs and Perennials: In the fall, plant spring-flowering bulbs like tulips, daffodils, crocuses, and hyacinths, as well as perennial flowers, shrubs, and trees, to establish root systems prior to winter dormancy.

Winter gardening tips:

1. Mulch around the base of perennial plants, shrubs, and trees to insulate roots, retain soil moisture, and protect against freeze-thaw cycles and winter damage.

2. Plan and Prepare: Use the winter months to plan next year's garden layout, research new plant varieties, order seeds, and stock up on gardening supplies in preparation for the upcoming growing season.

3. Maintain Tools and Equipment: Clean, sharpen, and oil gardening tools and equipment, such as pruners, shears, shovels, and hoes, and store them properly to prevent rust and extend their life.

4. Plant seeds indoors for early spring crops like tomatoes, peppers, eggplants, and herbs, using seed trays, grow lights, and heat mats to promote germination and seedling growth.

5. Feed Birds and Wildlife: During the winter months, install bird feeders, bird baths, and nesting boxes to support biodiversity and ecological balance in the garden. Following these seasonal gardening tips will help you optimize plant growth, manage garden tasks effectively, and have a successful and rewarding gardening experience all year. Stay informed, observe plants on a regular basis, and adjust gardening practices to accommodate seasonal changes, ensuring your garden's long-term health and productivity.

Spring Gardening Tasks

Spring is a vibrant time in the garden, when plants awaken from their winter dormancy and new growth appears. It's an excellent time to plant seeds, transplant seedlings, and prepare your garden for the growing season ahead.

Here are some essential spring gardening tasks to help you get your garden started:

1. Soil preparation: Begin by evaluating soil conditions, including pH and nutrient levels. Use compost, aged manure, or organic matter to improve soil fertility, structure, and drainage. Till or turn the soil to aerate and loosen compacted soil while removing weeds, rocks, and debris.

2. Planting: Sow seeds indoors for warm-season crops like tomatoes, peppers, eggplants, and squash. Once the soil is workable, sow cool-season crops like lettuce, spinach, radishes, carrots, peas, and beets directly into the garden. Place seedlings or nursery-grown plants in garden beds or containers, following spacing and planting guidelines.

3. Pruning and maintenance: Prune dormant trees, shrubs, and fruit trees to eliminate dead, damaged, or crossing

branches and promote healthy growth. Trim back perennial herbs, grasses, and ornamental plants to promote new growth and shape. Clean and sharpen garden tools such as pruners, shears, and shovels in preparation for the gardening season.

4. Weed Control: Hand-pull, hoe, or cultivate winter and emerging spring weeds to avoid competition with garden plants. Mulch around plants to control weed growth, retain soil moisture, and regulate soil temperature.

5. Pest and disease management: Keep an eye out for pests such as aphids, caterpillars, slugs, and snails on your plants and take appropriate action to control them. Inspect plants for signs of disease, such as fungal infections, powdery mildew, or leaf spots, and remove infected plant material immediately.

6. Fertilization: Use balanced fertilizers or organic amendments to provide essential nutrients to plants as they begin to grow in the spring. Add slow-release fertilizers or compost to planting holes or soil surfaces to encourage healthy root development and plant vigor.

7. Watering: Water newly planted seeds, seedlings, and transplants frequently to keep the soil evenly moist and

promote establishment. Keep track of soil moisture levels and adjust watering frequency and duration according to weather and plant requirements.

8. Plan and design: Spend time planning and designing your garden layout, including crop rotation, companion planting, and succession planting techniques. When arranging plants in garden beds or containers, take into account sunlight exposure, plant spacing, and growth habits. By completing these spring gardening tasks, you can lay the groundwork for a successful growing season and a plentiful harvest of fresh fruits, vegetables, herbs, and flowers all year. Stay organized, pay attention to plant needs, and enjoy the beauty and bounty of your spring garden.

Summer Gardening

Summer is a dynamic time in the garden, when plants thrive in warmth and sunlight and grow rapidly. However, it is also a season of challenges, including heat stress, water management, and pest control.

Here are some essential summer gardening tips to keep your garden healthy and productive:

1. Watering: Water deeply but infrequently to promote deep root growth and drought tolerance in plants. Water early in the morning or late in the afternoon to minimize evaporation and lower the risk of foliar diseases. Use drip irrigation, soaker hoses, or watering wands to deliver water directly to the root zone while reducing water waste.

2. Mulching: To conserve soil moisture, suppress weeds, and regulate soil temperature, spread a thick layer of organic mulch around plants, such as straw, wood chips, or compost. Replenish mulch as needed throughout the summer to ensure a consistent layer and maximum moisture and nutrient retention.

3. Fertilization: Feed plants on a regular basis with balanced fertilizers or organic amendments to replenish nutrients and promote rapid growth during the active growing season. Use liquid fertilizers or foliar sprays to promote rapid nutrient uptake and address nutrient deficiencies in plants exhibiting stress or nutrient imbalances.

4. Pest and Disease Management: Regularly inspect plants for signs of pests such as aphids, spider mites, whiteflies, and caterpillars, and take appropriate action to control infestations. To effectively manage pest populations, use integrated pest management (IPM) techniques like hand-picking, insecticidal soaps, neem oil, or biological controls. Monitor for signs of fungal diseases such as powdery mildew, blight, or rust, and ensure adequate air circulation, spacing, and sanitation to reduce disease pressure.

5. Shade and Protection: Shade heat-sensitive plants like lettuce, spinach, and Cole crops with shade cloth, row covers, or by planting them in the shadow of taller plants or structures. To protect plants from excessive heat, sunburn, or sunscald, provide temporary shade structures or use reflective mulch to deflect sunlight.

6. Harvesting and maintenance: Harvest fruits, vegetables, and herbs on a regular basis to ensure continuous production and avoid over-ripeness or spoilage. Deadhead flowers, remove spent blooms, and prune overgrown or leggy plants to stimulate new growth and extend flowering. Weed garden beds on a regular basis, replenish mulch, and remove debris to keep plants healthy and pest and disease pressure down.

7. Hydration and self-care: Stay hydrated and take breaks in hot weather to prevent heat exhaustion or dehydration while gardening. Wear sunscreen, protective clothing, and a wide-brimmed hat to protect yourself from the sun's harmful UV rays and avoid sunburn or heat-related illnesses. By following these summer gardening tips, you can keep your garden thriving during the hottest months of the year while enjoying a bounty of fresh produce, colorful blooms, and lush foliage all season long. Stay vigilant, stay hydrated, and savor the beauty and abundance of your summer garden.

Fall Gardening Chords

Fall is a transitional season in the garden, signaling the end of the growing season and preparing for winter dormancy. It's an important time to clean up the garden, harvest the last of the crops, and prepare plants for the winter months ahead.

Here are some important fall gardening chores that will keep your garden healthy and productive:

1. Harvesting: Harvest any remaining fruits, vegetables, and herbs before the first frost arrives. Collect seeds from annual plants to save and replant the following season. Keep harvested crops cool and dry, or preserve them by canning, freezing, or drying for long-term storage.

2. Cleaning and clearing: Clear garden beds and containers of spent plants, weeds, and debris to prevent overwintering pests and diseases. Remove dead or diseased foliage from perennials, herbs, and ornamental plants to improve air circulation and lower disease pressure. To prevent pathogen spread, clean and sanitize garden tools, pots, and equipment before storing them over the winter.

3. Soil preparation: Test soil pH and nutrient levels, and add organic matter, compost, or fertilizers as needed to replenish nutrients and improve soil fertility for the following growing season. Use a layer of organic mulch, such as straw, leaves, or compost, to protect soil from erosion, suppress weeds, and insulate plant roots from temperature changes.

4. Planting and transplanting: Grow cool-season crops like spinach, lettuce, kale, carrots, radishes, and garlic for the fall and winter harvests. Transplant perennials, shrubs, and trees while the soil is still warm to promote root development before winter dormancy.

5. Protection and Preparedness: To protect tender plants from frost damage, cover them with frost blankets, row covers, or cloches, or move them indoors if possible. Drain and winterize outdoor irrigation systems, hoses, and watering equipment to avoid freezing and damage during the cold season. Use mulch, burlap wraps, or protective covers to protect sensitive plants like roses, tender perennials, and newly planted trees from harsh winter weather.

6. Plan and design: Take the time to reflect on the previous growing season, assessing successes, challenges, and lessons

learned. Plan your garden layout, crop rotation, and planting schedule for the coming year, taking into account sunlight exposure, soil conditions, and plant compatibility.

7. Maintenance and organization: Maintain garden structures, pathways, and infrastructure by repairing fences, trellises, raised beds, and garden borders as necessary. Store garden supplies, tools, and equipment in a clean, dry location, and inventory seeds, bulbs, and gardening materials for the following season. Create a winter garden care schedule and calendar to help you stay organized and prioritize tasks for winter maintenance and garden preparation. By completing these fall gardening tasks, you can prepare your garden for the winter months and lay the groundwork for a successful and productive growing season the following year. Stay proactive and organized, and enjoy the beauty and tranquility of your garden as it enters the peaceful winter season.

Winter Garden Preparedness

Winter garden preparation is critical for protecting plants, soil, and structures from harsh weather and ensuring a successful start to the following growing season. Although gardening activity may slow down during the winter, there are still a few tasks to complete in order to keep a healthy and productive garden.

Here are some important winter garden preparation tips:

1. Clean up: Remove dead plants, weeds, and debris from garden beds, containers, and pathways to prevent pest and disease infestations. Cut back perennials and ornamental grasses to the ground, and prune back overgrown or damaged branches on trees and shrubs. To prevent pathogen spread, clean and sanitize garden tools, pots, and equipment before storing them over the winter.

2. Mulching: Cover garden beds with a thick layer of organic mulch like straw, leaves, or wood chips to insulate the soil, suppress weeds, and protect plant roots from freezing temperatures. Mulch around the base of tender perennials,

shrubs, and trees to protect them from frost damage and temperature fluctuations.

3. Protecting Plants Protect sensitive plants from freezing temperatures, frost, and windburn by using frost blankets, row covers, or burlap wraps. Cover the trunks of young trees and shrubs with tree wrap or burlap to prevent sunscald and frost cracking during cold weather. To protect potted plants and tender perennials from freezing temperatures, move them indoors or to a sheltered location like a greenhouse, porch, or garage.

4. Soil preparation: Test soil pH and nutrient levels, then amend with organic matter, compost, or fertilizer to replenish nutrients and improve soil structure for the following growing season. To prevent soil erosion and compaction, cover garden beds with mulch or plant cover crops to add organic matter and improve soil health.

5. Water and Irrigation: Drain and winterize outdoor irrigation systems, hoses, and watering equipment to avoid freezing and damage during the cold season. Water plants thoroughly before the ground freezes to ensure adequate

moisture for roots and reduce the risk of dehydration during the winter dormancy.

6. Structural maintenance: Examine garden structures such as fences, trellises, arbors, and raised beds for damage, rot, or instability, and repair or reinforce as necessary. Examine outdoor lighting, heating, and ventilation systems in greenhouses, cold frames, or hoop houses and make any necessary adjustments for winter conditions.

7. Planning and preparation: Take advantage of the quieter winter months to plan and design your garden layout, crop rotation, and planting schedule for the upcoming year. Order seeds, bulbs, and gardening supplies in advance and inventory existing supplies to ensure you have everything you need for spring planting.

8. Wildlife Management: Implement measures to deter wildlife such as deer, rabbits, rodents, and birds from damaging garden plants or accessing food sources during the winter. Install fencing, netting, or deterrents such as scare devices, motion-activated sprinklers, or repellents to protect crops and ornamental plants from wildlife damage.

CHAPTER 12

Advanced Gardening Techniques

Advanced gardening techniques include a variety of practices and strategies that go beyond basic gardening principles to optimize plant growth, maximize yields, and achieve exceptional garden results. These techniques often require a deeper understanding of plant biology, soil science, and ecological principles, as well as specialized skills and knowledge.

Here are some advanced gardening techniques to consider:

1. Soil Health and Management: Implement regenerative soil management practices such as no-till gardening, cover cropping, and composting to improve soil structure, fertility, and biological activity. Use soil testing and analysis to assess soil health and nutrient levels, and tailor amendments and fertilization strategies accordingly to optimize plant growth and productivity.

2. Crop rotation and companion planting: Develop comprehensive crop rotation plans to minimize soil depletion, pest buildup, and disease pressure by alternating crops with different nutrient needs and growth habits. Employ companion planting techniques to maximize plant health, pest resistance, and biodiversity by inter-planting compatible species that complement each other in terms of growth, nutrient uptake, and pest management.

3. Intensive Gardening Methods: Explore intensive gardening methods such as square foot gardening, raised bed gardening, and vertical gardening to maximize space efficiency, increase yields, and optimize resource use. Utilize techniques such as succession planting, intercropping, and trellising to make the most of limited garden space and extend the growing season for a diverse range of crops.

4. Hydroponics and Aquaponics: Experiment with hydroponic or aquaponics systems to grow plants in nutrient-rich water solutions or symbiotically with aquatic animals, respectively, without soil. Learn about different hydroponic growing methods, such as deep water culture, nutrient film

technique, and aeroponics, to cultivate plants in controlled environments and achieve rapid growth and high yields.

5. Season Extension and Microclimates: Extend the growing season by utilizing season extension techniques such as cold frames, hoop houses, row covers, or high tunnels to protect plants from frost and cold temperatures. Create microclimates within the garden by strategically placing plants near walls, fences, or thermal masses to capture and retain heat, shelter them from wind, or moderate temperature fluctuations.

6. Advanced Propagation Techniques: Master advanced propagation techniques such as grafting, air layering, tissue culture, and seed saving to propagate plants from specialized tissues, clones, or seeds and preserve genetic diversity. Experiment with hybridization, crossbreeding, or selection to develop new plant varieties with desired traits such as disease resistance, productivity, or flavor.

7. Organic Pest and Disease Management: Implement integrated pest management (IPM) strategies to control pests and diseases using natural enemies, biological controls, botanicals, and cultural practices while minimizing reliance

on synthetic pesticides. Practice advanced disease prevention techniques such as crop sanitation, crop rotation, resistant cultivar selection, and bio-fungicides to manage fungal, bacterial, and viral diseases effectively.

8. Precision Gardening and Technology: Embrace precision gardening techniques such as soil testing, pH monitoring, moisture sensors, and nutrient monitoring to optimize resource use, minimize waste, and achieve precise control over growing conditions. Explore emerging technologies such as remote sensors, automated irrigation systems, and smart gardening apps to streamline garden management, monitor plant health, and track environmental variables in real time. By incorporating advanced gardening techniques into your gardening repertoire, you can elevate your skills, expand your knowledge, and achieve greater success in cultivating healthy, productive, and sustainable gardens. Experiment with different techniques, adapt them to suit your specific growing conditions, and continue learning and exploring new approaches to take your gardening to the next level.

Companion Planting

Companion planting is a gardening technique that involves planting different species of plants together to enhance growth, productivity, and overall health. By strategically pairing plants based on their mutually beneficial relationships, gardeners can minimize pests, improve soil fertility, and increase yields.

Here's a detailed overview of companion planting:

1. Pest Management: Some plants generate natural substances or fragrances that repel pests or conceal the aroma of surrounding plants, minimizing the danger of insect infestations. For example: Marigolds (Tagetes spp.) generate a strong perfume that repels worms, aphids, and other insect pests, making them good partners for tomatoes, peppers, and brassicas. Alliums such as onions, garlic, and chives prevent pests like aphids, carrot flies, and cabbage worms when inter-planted with vulnerable crops like carrots, brassicas, and lettuce. Nasturtiums contain mustard oil chemicals that repel aphids, whiteflies, and squash bugs, making them good companions for cucumbers, squash, and tomatoes.

2. Attracting Beneficial Insects: Certain blooming plants attract beneficial insects such as bees, butterflies, and predatory insects that pollinate flowers, hunt pests, and help preserve ecological balance in the garden. For example: Umbelliferous herbs like dill, fennel, and cilantro attract beneficial insects such as ladybugs, lacewings, and hoverflies that feast on aphids, mites, and caterpillars, making them great partners for a wide range of garden crops. Yarrow (Achillea millefolium) and daisies attract pollinators such as bees and butterflies while supplying nectar and pollen for beneficial insects, promoting biodiversity and natural pest management in the garden.

3. Nutrient Accumulation and Soil Improvement: Some plants have deep root systems or specific nutrient absorption abilities that help them gather and recycle nutrients from the soil, increasing soil fertility and structure for surrounding plants. For example: Legumes such as peas, beans, and clover create symbiotic partnerships with nitrogen-fixing bacteria in their root nodules, enriching the soil with nitrogen and enhancing nitrogen availability for neighboring crops like leafy greens, tomatoes, and maize. Dynamic accumulators like comfrey, borage, and dandelion have deep

taproots that mine nutrients from the subsoil and accumulate minerals such as potassium, calcium, and phosphorus in their leaves, which may be utilized as nutrient-rich mulch or compost for other plants.

4. Space Utilization and Growth Habits: Companion planting helps gardeners optimize space use, increase yields, and limit competition by selecting plant combinations with complementary growth patterns and spatial requirements. For example: Tall, upright plants such as corn, sunflowers, and trellised cucumbers provide vertical support for vining crops like pole beans, peas, and squash, optimizing vertical growth area and boosting air circulation and light exposure. Ground-covering plants such as herbs, strawberries, and low-growing vegetables generate living mulch or weed-suppressing mats that shade the soil, preserve moisture, and prevent erosion while complementing taller crops and preserving space.

5. Succession planting and crop rotation: Companion planting may be integrated into succession planting and crop rotation programs to maximize plant health, prevent soil depletion, and discourage pests and diseases. For example:

Following heavy-feeding crops like tomatoes or cucumbers with nitrogen-fixing legumes such as beans or peas can restore soil nutrients and interrupt pest and disease cycles, boosting soil fertility and lowering the risk of soil-borne diseases. Rotating crops such as brassicas with alliums or legumes in various growing seasons can disrupt pest and disease cycles, regulate soil fertility, and increase overall garden health and production. Companion planting has various benefits for gardeners, including natural pest control, better soil fertility, enhanced biodiversity, and effective space management. By learning the concepts of companion planting and experimenting with different plant combinations, gardeners may construct resilient, balanced ecosystems that maintain healthy, productive gardens for years to come.

Crop Rotation

Crop rotation is a systematic process of growing various crops in the same area over successive seasons or years to enhance soil health, manage pests and diseases, and optimize crop yields. By rotating crops, gardeners may minimize soil depletion, reduce insect and disease burdens, and preserve long-term soil fertility.

Here's a full summary of crop rotation and its benefits:

1. Soil Health and Fertility: Different crops have variable nutritional requirements and interact with the soil in different ways. Crop rotation helps regulate soil fertility by alternating crops with various nutrient demands, minimizing the depletion of specific nutrients, and increasing overall soil health.

   Legumes such as peas, beans, and clover fix atmospheric nitrogen in their root nodules through symbiotic partnerships with nitrogen-fixing bacteria, enriching the soil with nitrogen and enhancing nitrogen availability for succeeding crops.

Deep-rooted crops like carrots, onions, and potatoes break up compacted soil, improve soil structure, and boost water and nutrient uptake, while shallow-rooted crops like lettuce, spinach, and radishes reach nutrients in the topsoil layers.

2. Pest and Disease Management: Continuous planting of the same crop in the same region can lead to the development of pests, illnesses, and soil-borne pathogens that target certain plant species. Crop rotation interrupts pest and disease cycles by depriving them of their preferred host plants and generating less favorable circumstances for their survival and reproduction. Plants from various botanical families have differential sensitivity to pests and diseases. Rotating crops among various plant families helps lessen the danger of reoccurring pest and disease issues by interrupting the continuous cycle of host plants and creating natural barriers to pest infestations. Certain crops emit natural substances called allele-chemicals that repel pests or prevent the growth of diseases in the soil, contributing to pest and disease control and increasing overall plant health.

3. Weed Control and Soil Conservation: Crop rotation can help suppress weeds and reduce weed pressure by disturbing weed germination and development cycles, shadowing the soil surface, and competing for resources such as water, sunshine, and nutrients. Cover crops such as clover, rye, and buckwheat may be used in crop rotation schemes to provide live mulch, reduce weeds, prevent erosion, and supply organic matter to the soil, boosting soil conservation and fertility.

4. Nutrient Cycling and Resource Management: Rotating crops with various nutrient requirements and growth patterns helps optimize nutrient cycling and resource usage in the garden, lowering the need for synthetic fertilizers and enhancing resource efficiency. Incorporating green manures, compost, and organic amendments into crop rotation programs provides organic matter to the soil, promotes microbial activity, and improves soil structure, water retention, and nutrient availability for succeeding crops.

5. Planning and Implementation: Develop a crop rotation plan based on the concepts of variety, succession, and

integration, taking into account aspects such as plant families, nutritional requirements, growth patterns, and pest and disease susceptibility. Divide the garden into discrete planting areas or blocks and rotate crops methodically within each area according to the specified rotation sequence, avoiding planting crops from the same family on the same site for successive seasons. Keep thorough records of crop rotations, planting dates, yields, and observations to track garden performance, detect patterns, and make educated decisions for future rotations and garden management.

By incorporating crop rotation into your gardening techniques, you can improve soil health, manage pests and diseases, and increase crop output in a sustainable and environmentally responsible manner. Experiment with alternative crop combinations and rotation sequences, adjust to your individual growing conditions, and enjoy the long-term advantages of healthy, resilient soils and numerous harvests.

Vertical Gardening

Vertical gardening is a gardening technique that involves growing plants vertically, utilizing structures such as trellises, arbors, fences, walls, or specialized vertical gardening systems. By exploiting vertical space, gardeners may optimize growing areas, boost crop yields, and create visually pleasing and space-efficient gardens.

Here's a full review of vertical gardening and its benefits:

1. Space Optimization: Vertical gardening helps gardeners make the most of limited space by growing plants vertically instead of spreading them out horizontally. This is especially excellent for urban gardens, tiny yards, balconies, patios, and other tight locations where horizontal space is limited. By adopting vertical structures such as trellises, arches, and vertical planters, gardeners may grow a varied range of plants vertically, including vining crops, climbing plants, and trailing ornamentals, while preserving ground area for other reasons.

2. Increased Growing Area: Vertical gardening enhances the available growth space by adding new growing surfaces and dimensions. This allows gardeners to grow more plants in the same footprint, boost crop diversity, and maximize garden output without extending the garden's physical footprint. By combining vertical features such as hanging baskets, wall-mounted planters, and tiered shelves, gardeners can construct multi-level gardens that suit a range of plant species and growing conditions, optimizing sunlight exposure and ventilation for maximum plant development.

3. Improved Air Circulation and Sunlight Exposure: Vertical gardening improves air circulation and sunlight penetration around plants, lowering the danger of fungal infections, insect infestations, and plant stress due to overcrowding and inadequate ventilation. Training plants to grow vertically on trellises or posts allows gardeners to better position plants, enhance light exposure to lower foliage, and promote air circulation inside the garden canopy, resulting in healthier, more productive plants.

4. Aesthetic appeal and design flexibility: Vertical gardens give visual interest, texture, and dimension to outdoor areas by forming vertical focal points, green walls, and living screens that improve the aesthetics of gardens, patios, and urban landscapes. Gardeners may construct and modify vertical gardens to their liking, using a range of plants, colors, textures, and structures to create one-of-a-kind garden displays that represent their particular flair and inventiveness.

5. Accessibility and Convenience: Vertical gardening makes it easier to access and maintain plants by eliminating the need to bend, crouch, or kneel when gardening. This is especially helpful for people with restricted mobility, physical limitations, or ergonomic issues. Vertical gardening, which raises plants to eye level or within an arm's reach, facilitates watering, trimming, harvesting, and pest monitoring, making gardening activities more accessible, efficient, and pleasurable for gardeners of all ages and abilities.

6. Sustainable gardening practices: Vertical gardening encourages sustainable growing methods by increasing

resource efficiency, reducing water consumption, and lowering environmental impact. Growing plants vertically allows gardeners to conserve water, decrease runoff, and improve irrigation efficiency by providing water directly to plant roots, reducing evaporation and soil moisture loss. Vertical gardens also allow you to recycle and repurpose items like pallets, pipes, containers, and recycled plastics to build your own vertical gardening structures, minimizing waste and supporting eco-friendly gardening methods. Overall, vertical gardening provides several advantages to gardeners, including space minimization, greater growing area, enhanced air circulation and sunshine exposure, aesthetic appeal, accessibility, and sustainability.

Gardeners that incorporate vertical planting techniques into their gardening repertoire may build attractive, productive, and space-efficient gardens that flourish in any environment. Experiment with various vertical gardening structures, plant combinations, and design concepts to unlock your creativity and maximize the possibilities of your vertical garden.

Hydroponics and Aquaponics

Hydroponics and aquaponics are new soilless gardening techniques that allow plants to thrive in nutrient-rich water solutions rather than soil, providing efficient and sustainable alternatives to standard soil-based gardening approaches. Both hydroponics and aquaponics use water-based systems to give nutrients to plants, but their approaches and system designs differ.

Here is a comprehensive introduction to hydroponics and aquaponics:

Hydroponics:

1. Nutrient Solutions: Hydroponic systems grow plants in water-based fertilizer solutions rich in critical elements including nitrogen, phosphorous, potassium, and micronutrients. Dissolving these nutrients in water and delivering them directly to plant roots eliminates the need for soil as a growth medium.

2. Growing Medium: Hydroponic systems use inert, soilless growth media like perlite, vermiculite, coconut coir, rock-wool, or clay pellets to support plant roots and

keep them stable. These media help plants stay in place while also allowing for proper root aeration, water retention, and nutrient uptake.

3. System types: Several varieties of hydroponic systems exist, including: Deep Water Culture (DWC): Plants are suspended in nutrient-rich water, with the roots submerged. The Nutrient Film Technique (NFT) involves continually flowing nutrient solution over plant roots in a shallow, recirculating film. Ebb and Flow (Flood and Drain): A nutrient solution is regularly injected into grow trays or containers and then emptied, giving plants intermittent watering cycles.

4. Water and nutrient management: To achieve maximum plant growth and health, hydroponic systems must carefully monitor water quality, pH levels, and fertilizer concentrations. Regularly examine and adjust pH levels to maintain the appropriate range for nutrient absorption. Nutrient solutions may need to be renewed, altered, or changed on a regular basis to avoid nutrient imbalances, algae growth, and nutrient shortages in plants.

Aquaponics:

1. Integrated systems: Aquaponics combines hydroponics and aquaculture, which is the production of aquatic creatures such as fish or shrimp in a symbiotic habitat. Beneficial bacteria convert fish waste products, typically ammonia, into nitrates in tanks or ponds.

2. Nutrient Cycling: In aquaponics systems, fish excrement acts as a natural fertilizer for plants, supplying critical nutrients including nitrogen, phosphorous, and potassium. Water from the fish tanks flows through grow beds or trays, where plants absorb nutrients and help filter out contaminants.

3. Beneficial bacteria: Beneficial bacteria play an important role in aquaponics systems by converting poisonous ammonia from fish waste into nitrites and ultimately nitrates, which plants may easily take as nutrients. This process, known as nitrification, improves water quality and promotes plant development.

4. Fish Selection: Aquaponics systems can support a wide range of freshwater fish species, including tilapia,

trout, catfish, and perch, as well as ornamental fish like koi or goldfish. Water temperature, pH requirements, stocking density, and intended harvest yield are all important considerations when selecting fish.

Advantages of hydroponics and aquaponics:

1. Water Efficiency: Hydroponic and aquaponics systems use water more effectively than traditional soil-based farming methods because water is recirculated and reused inside the system, reducing evaporation and runoff.

2. Space Optimization: Hydroponic and aquaponics systems may be used in a range of indoor and outdoor settings, making them ideal for cities, tiny spaces, and locations with limited access to arable land.

3. Year-round production: Hydroponic and aquaponics systems enable year-round production of fresh food and herbs, independent of seasonal or meteorological conditions. Controlled surroundings offer ideal growth

conditions for plants, resulting in regular harvests all year.

4. Sustainable practices: Hydroponics and aquaponics encourage sustainable farming methods by lowering soil erosion, water consumption, resource conservation, and the use of synthetic fertilizers and pesticides.

5. Educational Opportunities: Hydroponic and aquaponics systems provide tremendous teaching opportunities for students, enthusiasts, and gardeners who want to learn about plant biology, ecosystem dynamics, sustainable agriculture, and food production. While hydroponics and aquaponics have significant advantages, they require meticulous planning, maintenance, and monitoring to ensure maximum plant growth and system function

. Gardeners may develop flourishing, sustainable gardens by learning the fundamentals of hydroponics and aquaponics, as well as experimenting with different system designs, plant selections, and management strategies.

CHAPTER 13

Sustainable Gardening Practices

Sustainable gardening methods are ecologically conscious ways of gardening that seek to reduce negative environmental consequences, conserve natural resources, and enhance biodiversity and ecosystem health. Sustainable gardening includes a variety of strategies and philosophies that emphasize long-term land management while cultivating healthy, productive, and resilient gardens.

Here's an in-depth explanation of sustainable gardening practices:

1. Soil Health and Fertility: Use soil conservation and enhancement strategies like composting, mulching, and organic matter inclusion to create and sustain healthy, productive soil. Avoid using synthetic fertilizers, insecticides, and herbicides since they can harm soil bacteria, beneficial insects, and wildlife while also contributing to soil erosion and water pollution.

2. Water Conservation: usage of water-efficient irrigation solutions like drip irrigation, soaker hoses, or rainwater harvesting to reduce water waste and encourage effective water usage in the garden. Mulch garden beds with organic materials like straw, wood chips, or compost to keep soil wet, control weed development, and minimize evaporation from the soil surface.

3. Biodiversity and Habitat Creation: Plant a variety of native plants, flowers, and shrubs to attract pollinators, beneficial insects, and wildlife, as well as to establish habitat corridors for biodiversity in your garden. Use habitat elements like birdhouses, bee hotels, butterfly gardens, and wildlife-friendly plants to help native species and boost ecosystem resilience.

4. Organic pest and disease management: Use integrated pest management (IPM) tactics to control pests and illnesses, including natural predators, biological controls, cultural practices, and organic medicines like neem oil, insecticidal soaps, or botanical extracts. Rotate crops, use companion planting, and promote natural predators like ladybugs,

lacewings, and predatory insects to help control pest populations without using chemical pesticides.

5. Resource Efficiency and Waste Reduction: To reduce waste and save resources, recycle garden supplies like pots, containers, stakes, and trellises. Use eco-friendly gardening supplies, tools, and equipment made of recycled plastic, bamboo, or FSC-certified wood, and if feasible, opt for biodegradable or compostable options.

6. Energy Efficiency and Climate Resiliency: Use energy-efficient garden elements like passive solar design, windbreaks, and shadow structures to improve microclimates, minimize energy use, and buffer temperature extremes. Choose climate-appropriate plants and cultivars that are well-suited to local growth circumstances, need little maintenance, and are resistant to climate change and harsh weather occurrences.

7. Community Engagement and Education: Promote sustainable gardening concepts and practices by sharing information, resources, and best practices with fellow gardeners, neighbors, and community members via seminars, classes, or community gardening programs.

Encourage local food systems, community gardens, and urban agricultural initiatives that promote food security, social fairness, and environmental stewardship in your neighborhood. Gardeners who practice sustainable gardening may help to conserve and preserve the environment, promote biodiversity, and create resilient, healthy, and productive gardens that benefit people, plants, and the planet for future generations.

Water Conservation

Water conservation is the practice of using water in an efficient and responsible manner to reduce waste, maintain freshwater supplies, and protect the environment. Water conservation measures are critical in gardening because they keep plants healthy while minimizing water usage and supporting sustainable water management practices.

Here's a thorough summary of water-saving measures in gardening:

1. Efficient Irrigation System: Install water-efficient irrigation systems such as drip irrigation, soaker hoses, or micro-sprinklers to transport water directly to plant roots,

reducing evaporation and run-off. Use irrigation timers, sensors, or smart controllers to automate watering schedules, modify irrigation frequency and duration in response to weather conditions, and avoid overwatering.

2. Mulching: Cover garden beds with organic mulch such as wood chips, straw, or compost to preserve soil moisture, control weed development, and minimize evaporation. Mulching also regulates soil temperature, prevents erosion, and improves soil structure, resulting in healthier plant development and less water loss.

3. Watering Practices: Water plants deeply and rarely to foster deep root growth and drought tolerance, as opposed to shallow, frequent watering, which encourages shallow root systems and water waste. Water plants early in the morning or late in the evening to reduce water loss from evaporation and wind drift, and avoid watering during the warmest part of the day, when water is more likely to evaporate before reaching plant roots.

4. Soil preparation and improvements: Add organic matter to garden soil, such as compost, peat moss, or aged manure, to enhance soil structure, water retention, and drainage,

minimizing the need for regular irrigation. Use mulch, cover crops, or green manures to protect bare soil from erosion, retain soil moisture, and improve soil fertility, supporting healthy plant development and lowering runoff.

5. drought-tolerant plants: Select drought-tolerant or native plant species that are well-suited to the local environment and require little watering once established. Incorporate drought-tolerant ground coverings, ornamental grasses, succulents, and xeriscape plants into garden designs to create water-efficient landscapes that flourish with little water.

6. Harvesting rainwater: Collect and store rainwater from roof runoff, gutters, or downspouts in rain barrels, cisterns, or rain gardens to water garden plants, therefore decreasing dependency on municipal water supplies. Install rainwater harvesting systems with filters and diversion devices to efficiently collect, store, and distribute rainwater while reducing contamination and runoff pollution.

7. Soil Moisture Monitoring: Regularly monitor soil moisture levels with a soil moisture meter, probe, or simple hand-checking method to identify when plants want water and avoid overwatering or under watering. Modify irrigation

schedules and watering procedures based on soil moisture data, weather forecasts, and plant water requirements to guarantee plant health and water efficiency.

8. Water-Efficient Gardening Practices: Use water-saving gardening techniques like xeriscaping, which stresses water-wise landscaping concepts, native vegetation, and effective irrigation tactics to create low-maintenance, water-efficient landscapes. When designing and laying out a garden, go for water-efficient gardening methods such as container gardening, raised bed gardening, or vertical planting to maximize water consumption and decrease waste. By incorporating minimize water usage, protect freshwater resources, and promote sustainable water management practices by incorporating water conservation methods into their gardens.

Adopting water-saving practices not only conserves water but also lowers water costs, decreases environmental impact, and produces robust, drought-resistant landscapes that flourish in shifting climates.

Soil Health Preservation

Soil health preservation is the technique of preserving and improving soil's biological, physical, and chemical properties in order to promote healthy plant development, biodiversity, and ecosystem function. Healthy soil is critical for sustainable agriculture, food security, and environmental protection because it promotes nutrient cycling, water retention, carbon sequestration, and plant production.

Here's a full summary of soil health preservation practices:

1. Soil Testing and Analysis: Conduct frequent soil testing to determine soil pH, nitrogen levels, organic matter content, and soil texture, which will provide useful information for soil management and fertility planning. Use soil test findings to alter pH, balance nutrient levels, and adapt fertilizer applications to meet the individual needs of crops and plants, reducing nutrient imbalances and increasing nutrient availability.

2. Organic matter management: Add organic matter to the soil to increase soil structure, water retention, nutrient cycling, and microbial activity. Examples include compost,

aged manure, cover crops, and green manures. Composting converts organic waste from the garden, kitchen, or yard into nutrient-rich compost, which improves soil fertility, encourages beneficial soil organisms, and decreases the need for synthetic fertilizers.

3. Minimal soil disturbance: prevent soil disturbance using measures like no-till or limited tillage, which help protect soil structure, prevent erosion, and maintain soil organic matter levels. Use conservation tillage techniques like strip-tillage or zone-tillage to disrupt only a piece of the soil surface while leaving the bulk undisturbed, minimizing soil erosion and boosting water penetration.

4. Crop rotation and cover cropping: Use crop rotation to diversify plant species, interrupt pest and disease cycles, and replenish soil nutrients by using legumes or green manure crops. Plant cover crops like clover, rye, or vetch during fallow seasons or in between cash crops to prevent soil erosion, reduce weeds, fix nitrogen, and enhance soil structure and fertility.

5. Controlling soil erosion: Use erosion control techniques such as contour planting, terracing, mulching, or vegetative

buffers to reduce soil erosion, sediment runoff, and nutrient loss in agricultural areas. Maintain vegetative cover in the form of permanent plants, grassed rivers, windbreaks, or riparian buffers to stabilize soil, decrease surface runoff, and safeguard water quality in surrounding bodies.

6. Soil Amendments and Nutrient Management: Use organic soil amendments like bone meal, rock phosphate, or gypsum to replenish soil nutrients, raise soil pH, and improve nutrient availability to plants. Use nutrient management strategies like precision fertilization, split applications, or fertigation to increase fertilizer efficiency, limit nutrient runoff, and minimize environmental effects.

7. Soil biology and microbial activity: Improve soil biology and microbial variety by providing habitat and food for beneficial soil creatures, including earthworms, fungi, bacteria, and microorganisms. Avoid excessive use of synthetic pesticides, herbicides, and fungicides, which can kill beneficial soil organisms and alter soil food webs, jeopardizing soil health and ecosystem function.

8. Soil Conservation Planning and Education: Create complete soil conservation plans that cover erosion control,

nutrient management, water quality preservation, and sustainable land use practices based on individual soil types and landscape circumstances. Inform farmers, gardeners, landowners, and policymakers on the value of soil health preservation, sustainable soil management techniques, and the significance of healthy soils in promoting food security, environmental resilience, and ecosystem services.

Gardeners, farmers, and land managers who prioritize soil health preservation measures may increase soil fertility, productivity, and resilience while also safeguarding natural resources, fostering biodiversity, and minimizing environmental degradation. Sustainable soil management approaches improve agricultural output while simultaneously reducing climate change, conserving water, and ensuring ecosystem sustainability, resulting in healthier, more resilient landscapes for future generations.

Integrated Pest Management

Integrated Pest Management (IPM) is a comprehensive pest management method that focuses on preventive, monitoring, and control measures to reduce pest impact while minimizing threats to human health, beneficial creatures, and the environment. IPM combines a variety of pest management strategies, including biological, cultural, mechanical, and chemical approaches, to successfully manage pest populations and avoid pest damage in a sustainable and ecologically friendly way.

Here's a comprehensive review of integrated pest management:

1. Pest Identification and Monitoring: Conduct frequent scouting, observation, and trapping to determine pest numbers, distribution, and damage levels in the garden or agricultural areas. Use field guides, identification keys, and pest monitoring instruments, including sticky traps, pheromone traps, and insect nets, to identify pest species and follow population dynamics over time.

2. Cultural practices: Use cultural techniques, including crop rotation, sanitation, and plant spacing, to lessen pest pressure, interrupt insect life cycles, and create unfavorable circumstances for pest growth and reproduction. Select pest-resistant plant types, companion plantings, and trap crops that are less vulnerable to pest damage and act as natural pest deterrents.

3. Biological Control: Introduce natural enemies, predators, or parasites that feed on pest organisms in order to reduce pest populations and offer long-term, sustainable pest management. Provide habitat, food supplies, and shelter in your garden or agricultural environment to attract beneficial insects such as ladybugs, lacewings, predatory mites, and parasitic wasps.

4. Mechanical and physical controls: Remove or exclude pests from the garden or agricultural fields using mechanical and physical control methods such as handpicking, pruning, traps, or barriers. Use physical barriers like row covers, netting, or screens to shield plants from pests while still allowing ventilation, sunshine, and pollinator access.

5. Chemical Control: As a last option, use chemical pesticides sparingly and carefully to eliminate specific pests while limiting their impact on non-target creatures, beneficial insects, and environmental resources. Select the least toxic, low-risk pesticide formulations, such as insecticidal soaps, horticultural oils, or botanical insecticides, and follow the label directions and suggested application rates.

6. Monitoring and decision-making: Regularly monitor pest populations, crop health, and environmental variables to determine the efficacy of pest management measures and make educated pest control decisions. Using economic thresholds, pest forecast models, and risk assessment tools, identify when and where pest management activities are necessary based on pest population dynamics, crop value, and probable yield loss.

7. Record-keeping and evaluation: Keep thorough records of pest monitoring data, pest management activities, pesticide applications, and outcomes to track pest trends, assess control strategies, and enhance long-term IPM decision-making. Assess the effectiveness of IPM tactics based on

insect suppression, crop production, economic returns, environmental impact, and social acceptability, and alter management practices as necessary to maximize pest control outcomes. Gardeners, farmers, and land managers can effectively manage pest populations, reduce reliance on chemical pesticides, and promote sustainable pest control practices that protect human health, beneficial organisms, and the environment by incorporating a variety of pest management tactics and strategies into a comprehensive IPM approach.

IPM focuses on proactive, preventative methods and adaptive management tactics to reduce insect damage, maximize agricultural yields, and promote resilient, healthy ecosystems for future generations.

Composting and Recycling

Composting and recycling are important techniques in sustainable gardening and waste management because they help minimize organic waste, increase soil fertility, and promote environmental sustainability. Composting is the process of decomposing organic materials such as food scraps, yard waste, and other biodegradable materials into nutrient-rich compost, whereas recycling is the collection and processing of recyclable materials such as paper, plastic, glass, and metal for reuse or repurposing.

Here's a full breakdown of composting and recycling:

Composting:

1. Organic waste collection: Gather organic items, including fruit and vegetable scraps, coffee grounds, eggshells, yard trimmings, leaves, grass clippings, and shredded paper, for composting. Avoid composting meat, dairy, oils, fats, pet waste, and damaged plant materials since these may attract pests, emit aromas, or harbor diseases.

2. Composting Process: Layer organic materials in a compost bin, pile, or container, alternating between green

(high nitrogen) items like kitchen wastes and grass clippings and brown (high carbon) materials like dried leaves, straw, or shredded paper. Keep the compost pile wet but not soggy, and turn or aerate it on a regular basis to encourage oxygenation and decomposition, which will speed up the composting process. Keep track of compost temperature, moisture levels, and decomposition progress to guarantee the best conditions for microbial activity and organic matter breakdown.

3. Compost Maintenance: Keep track of compost temperature, moisture levels, and decomposition progress to guarantee the best conditions for microbial activity and organic matter breakdown. Turn or aerate the compost pile on a regular basis to mix materials, supply oxygen, and encourage even decomposition, which will speed up the composting process and prevent anaerobic situations.

4. Compost Use: When compost has decomposed completely and resembles black, crumbly soil, it is suitable for use as a nutrient-rich soil supplement, mulch, or top dressing in the garden, flower beds, or container plants. Mix compost into garden soil to enhance soil structure, water

retention, nutrient availability, and microbial activity, promoting plant development and minimizing the need for synthetic fertilizers.

Recycling:

1. Material Separation: Separate recyclable items like paper, cardboard, plastics, glass, aluminum, and metal cans from non-recyclable garbage to make recycling easier to collect and process. Before recycling, rinse and sanitize recyclable containers to remove any food residue, labels, or pollutants to guarantee high-quality materials for processing.

2. Recycling Collection: Enroll in curbside recycling programs run by local municipalities or waste management businesses to have recyclable goods collected from your house or company for processing. If curbside recycling is not available in your region, drop recyclable goods off at approved recycling centers, transfer stations, or drop-off sites.

3. Recycling Processing: Recyclable items are transported to recycling facilities, where they are sorted, cleaned, and processed into raw materials or secondary products used to

make new products. Paper, cardboard, plastic bottles, glass containers, and aluminum cans are sorted, baled, and delivered to factories, where they are recycled into new paper goods, plastic bottles, glass containers, and aluminum cans.

4. Recycled Product Use: Buy recycled items, such as recycled paper, plastic lumber, glass containers, or aluminum cans, to help recycle markets and encourage the usage of recycled resources. Complete the recycling loop by recycling products and packaging materials at the end of their life cycle to save resources, decrease waste, and lessen environmental impact.

Composting and recycling allow individuals to decrease trash, save resources, and promote environmental sustainability in their communities. Composting organic materials diverts trash from landfills, lowers greenhouse gas emissions, and generates useful compost for soil enrichment and plant development. Recycling recyclable materials helps to conserve natural resources, reduce energy consumption, and promote the creation of new goods from recycled materials, all of which contribute to a circular economy and sustainable resource management.

Conclusion

Finally, sustainable gardening methods like composting and recycling are critical for encouraging environmental stewardship, conserving natural resources, and cultivating healthy, resilient ecosystems. Composting in garden management converts organic waste into nutrient-rich compost, which improves soil fertility, increases plant growth, and reduces dependency on synthetic fertilizers. Similarly, recycling recyclable items diverts trash from landfills, conserves resources, and encourages the development of new goods from recycled materials, all of which contribute to a circular economy and sustainable resource management.

Furthermore, sustainable gardening strategies such as water conservation, soil health preservation, integrated pest control, and biodiversity conservation are critical for keeping gardens healthy and productive while reducing environmental impact and improving ecosystem resilience. Gardeners may create vibrant, sustainable landscapes that promote biodiversity, offer habitat for wildlife, and contribute to community and ecosystem health and well-being by using a holistic approach to gardening that incorporates a variety of methods and approaches. To summarize, composting and recycling are essential components of sustainable gardening, demonstrating the necessity of waste reduction, resource conservation, and environmental sustainability in garden management.

Individuals who adopt sustainable gardening techniques and concepts may have a positive influence on the environment, improve the beauty and productivity of their gardens, and encourage others to establish a deeper connection with the natural world. Together, we can make the world a more sustainable place for future generations.

www.ingramcontent.com/pod-product-compliance
Lightning Source LLC
Chambersburg PA
CBHW051555250726
48653CB00004BA/1166